SERVE THE PEOPLE

SERVE THE PEOPLE

*Observations on Medicine in
the People's Republic of China*

VICTOR W. SIDEL
and
RUTH SIDEL

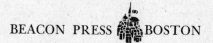

BEACON PRESS BOSTON

Copyright © 1973 by Josiah Macy, Jr. Foundation

First published as a Beacon Paperback in 1974
by arrangement with the Josiah Macy, Jr. Foundation

Beacon Press books are published under the auspices
of the Unitarian Universalist Association

Published simultaneously in Canada by Saunders of Toronto, Ltd.

All rights reserved

Printed in the United States of America

9 8 7 6 5 4 3 2 1

Library of Congress Cataloging in Publication Data

Sidel, Victor W
    Serve the people.
    Reprint of the ed. published by Josiah Macy Foundation,
New York, in series: Macy Foundation series on medicine and
public health in China.
    Bibliography: pp. 299–307.
    1. Medical care — China.   2. Medicine — China.
I. Sidel, Ruth, joint author.   II. Title.
III. Series: Josiah Macy Jr. Foundation, New York. The
Macy Foundation series on medicine and public health in China.
[RA527.S5   1974]   362.1'0951   74–6185
ISBN 0–8070–2175–X

为中美两国人民之间的友谊

To the Friendship between the Chinese and American Peoples

Contents

Tables, Figures, and Appendices

Preface

Victor W. Sidel, a physician specializing in community medical care, and Ruth Sidel, a psychiatric social worker, are a husband-and-wife team uniquely qualified to observe and analyze medical programs. They had the rare good fortune to visit the People's Republic of China for this purpose on two occasions in 1971 and 1972. The second visit gave them an opportunity to validate and expand their earlier observations, which have been reported extensively. Their deep commitment to studies on China not only made them most welcome guests but also afforded superb opportunities for fact finding.

Their observations on medical care are enhanced by their previous studies in other countries which afford interesting opportunities for comparative analyses of, for example, the Russian feldsher and the barefoot doctor in China.

It is clear from the reports of the Sidels and others that since 1950 China has accomplished massive and effective reforms in medical care; she has also established philosophies and patterns that should be studied carefully by all countries.

We hope this book will serve as a comprehensive description of medical care in China today.

JOHN Z. BOWERS, M.D.
President
Josiah Macy, Jr. Foundation

August 27, 1973

Introduction

THE initial opportunity to gather the material presented in this report arose as a result of an invitation from the Chinese Medical Association (CMA) to visit the People's Republic of China (PRC) as its guests during September and October 1971. Independently invited at approximately the same time were Mary and E. Grey Dimond, provost for the health sciences, University of Missouri, Kansas City; Helen and Samuel Rosen, professor emeritus of otology, Mount Sinai School of Medicine, New York City; and Ina and Paul Dudley White of Boston. Their visits overlapped somewhat with ours.*

The privilege of being among the first visitors from the United States to the PRC in twenty-two years came about in part because we have long been interested in medical and social services in other countries and their implications for the United States. When the American table tennis team's visit to China in April 1971 seemed to open the door to American visitors, we immediately wrote to the Ottawa Embassy of the PRC requesting a visa. Like thousands of others, we received no reply.

Then, in May, Professor Arthur Galston of Yale and Professor Ethan Signer of MIT received visas for the PRC, thus becoming the first American scientists to visit China since shortly after 1949. On his return, Galston, with whom one of us had been associated in analysis and criticism of the use of chemical weapons in Vietnam by the United States, wrote a letter on our behalf to Dr. Kuo Mo-jo, President of the Chinese Academy of Sciences, whom he had met in Peking. Three months later, on September 1, Galston received a reply inviting us to come to China as guests

---

* A number of the reports written by these visitors and about the visits are listed in the Bibliography of this volume.

1

of the CMA. We spent from September 20 to October 14 in the PRC; a list of the institutions and the people we visited is given in Appendix A.

One year later, following considerable study, lecturing, and writing on China, we were invited by the CMA to return, this time with our two sons—Mark, age fourteen, and Kevin, age thirteen. This visit was somewhat longer, from September 4 to October 5, 1972; the cities and institutions we visited are given in Appendix B. As in our first visit, all of our expenses in China were paid by the CMA, and we were accompanied by CMA guides and interpreters throughout our visit.

Finally, we had an opportunity to discuss our observations and to gain further insight through conversations with members of the CMA delegation that visited the United States in October 1972; the members of the delegation are listed in Appendix C. We had the privilege of acting as co-hosts to the delegation (along with the Institute of Medicine of the National Academy of Sciences and the American Medical Association, and the Dimonds, Rosens, and Whites) and accompanied it through most of its visit. We had especially fruitful discussions with Dr. Hsu Chia-yu, who had accompanied us throughout our first visit to China, had spent several days with us on our second visit, and whom we now regard as our *lao pengyou,* "old friend."

The Limitations of the Visits

In the course of our first visit we spent a week in Shanghai, China's largest city; ten days in Peking, the capital and second largest city; and several days in each of two smaller cities, Kwang-chow (Canton) and Hangchow. We also had an opportunity to visit the rural areas surrounding these cities. During our second visit we returned to Kwangchow, Peking, and Shanghai and their surrounding areas, and had the privilege of traveling to Shih-kiachwang, Yenan, Sian, and the famous Tachai Production Brigade. In the course of these visits we had ample opportunity to discuss various aspects of medical care with officials of the CMA, with officials, teachers, and students at six of China's medical schools, and with health workers and patients in hospitals, health stations, and other urban medical facilities. In the rural areas we visited county hospitals and communes, production brigades, and production teams, talked with their medical personnel and observed their facilities. A wealth of material was generously shared with us. Most important, we were able to observe directly the functioning of some aspects of the medical care system.

It must be stated at the outset, however, that our observations on medicine in China suffer from limitations of time, logistics, competence, and bias. Two months is too short a period for an extensive study of almost any aspect of a foreign culture, let alone areas as broad as we attempted to review. Our interests and observations ranged from neighborhood health stations to acupuncture anesthesia, and from preschool education to the role of the aged. Logistically the visitor in a country such as China is dependent on his hosts, and although our requests to visit certain types of institutions and people were almost invariably granted, our intensive investigative efforts were of necessity limited to the specific facilities and personnel chosen for us by our hosts. While we have studied medical care and social services in other countries such as the Soviet Union and Great Britain, our range of competence involved little background knowledge of China and almost no knowledge of the Chinese language. Finally, while we made every effort to be as objective as possible, we clearly took biases and preconceptions with us; some of these are detailed below.

One additional point of caution must be raised. Many analysts of Chinese affairs have commented on the fact that Chinese spokesmen sometimes present their ideals as realities, even if the ideals have not yet been realized. This must not be viewed as mendacity or as the construction of a "Potemkin village"—all facade and no substance behind it. It is much more subtle: It is an attempt to inspire the visitor, and themselves, with a vision of what life should be like. Apart from direct observations, therefore, it is sometimes difficult for the short-term visitor to sort out the prodigious feats already accomplished from the even greater accomplishments that are earnestly sought.

What follows must thus be viewed as fragmentary, and should, as should any "instant expert's" report, be read with skepticism. For example, we mention only in passing many important elements of medicine in China—such as their success in replanting severed limbs—which we did not have an opportunity to observe or to discuss in detail while there. Nonetheless it seems important to record these personal observations on medicine in China so that they may raise questions and provide a starting point for further exploration. It is in this spirit, rather than as a definitive document on the topic, that this monograph is presented.

Preconceptions and Observations

It is important to attempt to spell out some of our preconceptions because frequently one sees what one expects to see. Nowhere has this truism been stated more pointedly than in the bit of doggerel that Newsholme and Kingsbury quoted in *Red Medicine,* the report of their 1933 visit to the Soviet Union:

> The sights that X selected
> Bore out what he expected—
> Great factories rising;
> An enthusiasm surprising
> For welfare and education;
> A New World in formation
> Much better than the Old—
> Just as he had foretold.

> Mr. Y saw what he expected—
> Breakdowns in transportation;
> A growing indignation
> With the Communist oppression;
> A steady retrogression
> To chaos, bloody and red—
> Just as he had always said.

Our bias that there is much that needs improvement in the American health care system—and in American society in general —unquestionably led us to look with friendly interest on a system of social and health services that had been reported to have produced almost unbelievable progress in just two decades. But although this bias was a positive one many of our other preconceptions were negative. Although we knew that most of the people lived in rural areas, our image of China was one of poor, teeming, jangling cities. We expected, too, a highly regimented society with an air of worship of Mao Tse-tung, and one of monotony unrelieved by variety. Although we knew that the Cultural Revolution had changed some things, we expected to be put off by a managerial and Communist Party elite. We expected also to find an overwhelming, and to us highly distasteful, military presence.

What we actually found was very different. China is predominantly rural, and our lasting impression is of a vast countryside, green and heavily planted. Its cities are mostly carless, clean, and calm, with people showing little or no sign of boredom, cynicism, or irritability. Its great masses of courteous, enormously hardworking people, surprised us immediately as we realized that the general uniformity of their dress in no way makes them either faceless or anonymous. Indeed, we grew more sensitive to faces and their expressions than to the styles of clothing and manner that usually stand out among Westerners.

We began to explore China through our Chinese hosts. We found a country with a deep sense of mission and history, a nation trying all at one time to be daringly experimental, uncompromisingly doctrinaire, and unconstrainedly pragmatic. In the last few years China has become "democratic" and egalitarian in an antielitist, antihierarchical way that differentiates it from both the Soviet and American patterns. And above all it has become the center of some extremely strong beliefs about the individual and the world—that the highest purpose of the individual is selfless service to the people; that the people working together can achieve almost any goal; and that involvement in politics should be total, that it should in fact suffuse every aspect of life.

Just how seriously many Chinese take those beliefs, and how those beliefs, with their widespread literal acceptance, now form the intellectual keystone of the country's huge structure of medical and social services, was demonstrated to us daily if not hourly in 1971, as spokesman after spokesman—in hospitals, kindergartens, factories, communes, and research institutes—expressed to us the importance in their work of Mao Tse-tung and his Thought.

The attitude toward Mao is exemplified by a story told us by R. J. David Turnbull, an Australian general practitioner and senator, who visited China during the height of the Cultural Revolution. At a Shanghai hospital Dr. Turnbull was shown a man who had had a severed right arm replanted, a feat of which both the patient and his doctors were justifiably proud. The patient lifted a pail of water with his right arm and said, "Thanks to Chairman Mao, I can now lift this pail of water again." "Just a minute," said the Australian, "Why don't you thank your surgeon here instead of Chairman Mao?" The surgeon interrupted: "I was the son of a poor peasant family. In the Old China I could never have dreamed of becoming educated as a doctor. That I was able to do so, and was therefore here to sew this man's arm back on, is indeed due to the revolution made for us by Chairman Mao."

As we heard it, part of the reverence for Mao as a man is that symbolically he represents the revolution and the changes it has brought about in people's lives. But the reverence for Mao's Thought is of a much deeper nature and pervades the entire society. In fact, of Mao's many titles—"leader," "chairman," "helmsman," and the like—the one likely to survive is that of "teacher," a kind of latter-day Confucius whose greatest genius lay not in military strategy and tactics, though he did those well enough; not in government organization, in which his record has not been perfect by any means; and not in the day-to-day management of current affairs, which it is unlikely that he now does—his genius was in laying out a set of principles, based in part on the traditions of the past and on theories of the future, for a society to follow.

Maoist principles appear in every element of Chinese society. A leading one is found in "Serve the People," the first of Mao's "Constantly Read Articles," according to which individual merit is measured by selflessness and willingness to work for common goals. Thus political attitude has become important in all aspects of the society, including medical care. Another principle is the lesson of "The Foolish Old Man Who Removed the Mountains,"

Mao's "Third Constantly Read Article," * which is that the mass of people working in concert can move mountains. To take an example from health care, by mobilizing mass movements, social diseases such as venereal disease, drug addiction, or alcoholism can be conquered. By the time of our 1972 visit these articles and other visible evidence of Mao were much less omnipresent, but their power and influence seemed undiminished.

Another important principle, strengthened by the Cultural Revolution, is the Chinese faith in learning by doing, and in learning precisely what is needed, no more, no less, to do any given job. Perhaps crucial to this whole complex edifice is a constant effort to combat rivalry and careerism and to foster cooperation and teamwork. The People's Liberation Army, for example, is visible everywhere, but in an essentially helpful role— part civilian conservation corps, part VISTA, part public health service, part management consultant. No doubt other army members or even the same ones we saw at other times and places are practicing marching or whatever it is that armies do to prepare for, or as the Chinese put it, "against," war. But their one highly visible function, in the tradition of Mao's Eighth Route Army, is to render service.

In almost all of our meetings with professional health and other service people, "paraprofessionals" and "nonprofessionals" were present and encouraged to speak up without any formality or awe of authority. A medical professor, the head of a commune hospital, a barefoot doctor, a midwife—each exhibited a calm assurance that left us with a strong impression of comradeship and a genuine attempt at equality.

Finally, one of our major preconceptions in 1971 was that although we would find the hospitality for which the Chinese are famous, it would be tempered by the fact that we were Americans. In actuality, the friendliness and hospitality that was accorded to us was one of the most memorable aspects of our visits to China. This was true not only of our hosts in the

* The "Second Constantly Read Article," an essay in memory of Dr. Norman Bethune, is reprinted in full in Appendix D.

CMA who did everything to make our trips comfortable, pleasurable, and productive, but of the staff in the hotels, communes, factories, and hospitals we visited. We were greeted at each airport or train station by a group of staff members and physicians of the local branch of the CMA, and for the most part this group toured all facilities with us in their respective cities. All were eager to answer our questions and repeatedly explained those things we did not understand. When we saw slides on Norman Bethune used in a kindergarten class to teach internationalism, self-reliance, and selflessness, and said we would very much like to have a set, our hosts scoured Peking and Shanghai and presented the slides to us as a gift. They laboriously helped us to learn some Chinese phrases and to read some of the posters, never showing a hint of impatience. They repeatedly reminded us of the traditional friendship between the Chinese and American peoples, which they hoped would be renewed and strengthened by increasing contact.

ECHOES OF THE PAST

The organization of health care services in any nation can be fully understood only when viewed against the backdrop of its history. One reason is obvious: Current patterns must be compared to those in the recent and less recent past, so that progress can be measured and reasonable projections made for the near future. But in China a second reason is especially important: the necessity for an understanding of the impact of the past upon the present. In no other society has so great an effort been made to remember the past, to remedy its errors, and, most important, to build upon its strengths.

Many "China watchers" have commented on the role of China's history in its current policies. Much has been made, for example, of the ancient concept of China as the Middle Kingdom, the center of the world to which other nations came to *koutou* (the source, of course, of our word kowtow), and of the impact of this concept of China's past centrality on its present foreign policies. Examples of the Chinese attempt to remember and learn from their past are everywhere, from the restoration of the

Ming Tombs, where there are charts showing how much rice for starving peasants might have been provided by the riches and labor spent in their construction, to a special role for elderly people, who visit the schools regularly to teach about the "bitter past." In medicine, examples from the past to be emulated or to be avoided also abound, from the "treasurehouse" of traditional Chinese medicine to the "elitism" of the Peking Union Medical College.

But in addition to being seen against the backdrop of the past, health care services must be viewed against the setting of the present, again for at least two reasons. The first is that medical care and preventive medicine are never practiced—and can therefore never be evaluated—in a vacuum, but must always be seen as relative to the specific social and medical needs of the people they seek to serve. These needs must be understood if the goals, successes, and failures of the medical care system are to be understood. The second reason, again especially true of China, is that social forces play a major role in shaping medical care patterns, which are hard to understand without some knowledge of the forces impinging on them.

China today is still in the throes of major social upheaval. The advent of Communist political control was as recent as 1949; and the Great Proletarian Cultural Revolution that began in 1966 was in many ways still going on in 1971. The response to many of our questions about medical care organization, education, and evaluation was that the "struggle, criticism, and transformation" of the Cultural Revolution was not yet complete and that new patterns had not yet stabilized. By 1972 the atmosphere seemed to have changed considerably; the Cultural Revolution, while not yet over, had at least entered a new phase.

Thus the system of medical care in China must be seen as part of still changing patterns of a society in flux. The pendulum set in motion by the Cultural Revolution was still swinging at the time of our visits. In fact to us the most exciting feature of a study of medicine in China is the insights it gives into the interaction between past and present and between health services and other elements of social change. Therefore, although it would have been tempting—and much simpler—to limit this account to the things we actually saw and heard, it will be necessary to include in each chapter a limited amount of material about the past, and about elements of the present society that we did not personally explore.

TRANSLITERATION AND TRANSLATION

The transliteration (Romanization) of Chinese words used in this volume, with the exception of the names of people and places, is based whenever possible on the relatively new *pinyin* (Chinese phonetic alphabet), the system in official use in the People's Republic. For the transliteration of people's names, and for some other words and phrases, in general the Chinese continue to use elements of the older Wade-Giles (Yale) system. Thus our 1971 interpreter's name, pronounced "Shoo" in English, would be rendered as "Xu" in *pinyin;* but he himself, and official PRC agencies, still prefer to write it, when they write in English, as "Hsu," according to the Wade-Giles system. For places, the "post office names" continue to be used; for example, although "Beijing" is the *pinyin,* and "Pei-ching" the Wade-Giles transliteration, both Americans and Chinese consistently transliterate the name of China's capital as "Peking." There are numerous other inconsistencies in current English transliteration in China. For example, in Kwangchow the name of our hotel (the Eastern) is transliterated on its own stationery as "Tung Fang," whereas the rendering in *pinyin* should be "Dong Fang," and the name of the Dr. Sun Yat-sen Medical College is given as "Chung-shan" rather than "Zhongshan." We, too, have made no attempt at complete consistency in transliteration.

The translations into English are whenever possible, those given by our Chinese hosts or those used in Chinese publications. A few terms were translated for us by our hosts in more than one way. For example, the name of the organization which invited us was translated into English by different interpreters as All-China Medical Association, China Medical Association, and Chinese Medical Association; we have arbitrarily chosen to use one form only, in this case the last.

A special problem arises with translation of the names of the medicines used in China. For traditional Chinese medicines, the best that can be done until English-language formularies are available is to simply transliterate the Chinese name. For Western-type medicines, most of which are now manufactured in China, the Chinese often use what would in the United States be regarded as the brand name rather than the generic name. For example, the drug whose generic name in the United States is chlordiazepoxide hydrochloride is given on bottle labels and by interpreters in China as "librium," its Roche Laboratories brand name. Even the handbooks of drugs for doctors and for barefoot doctors, which often list the Romanized equivalents, call the drug "librium." In other instances, what we would consider the generic name is used. For example, chlorphenira-mine maleate is known as such, rather than by the Schering Corporation's brand name, Chlor-trimeton, by which it is far better known in the United States. When drug names are used in the following chapters we will therefore use the name by which the drug is commonly known in China; if that happens to be the brand name used in the United States, we will place it in quotation marks and supply its generic name in parentheses.

The Land, the People, and the Economy

Although it is impossible in a few introductory pages to cover adequately topics on each of which volumes have been written (see the Bibliography), it is equally impossible in our view to discuss a nation's health services without at least a brief description of the people the services are designed to serve and the conditions of their life. China's mainland territory, as may be seen in Figure 1, covers a land area of 3,692,000 square miles, about 20 per cent greater than that of the United States excluding Alaska (3,089,000 square miles), and almost exactly the same size as the United States if Alaska is included (3,675,000 square miles). In latitude China is situated very similarly on its side of the earth as is the United States almost exactly on the other side. The climate of most of China is therefore not very different from that of parts of the United States, with the excep-

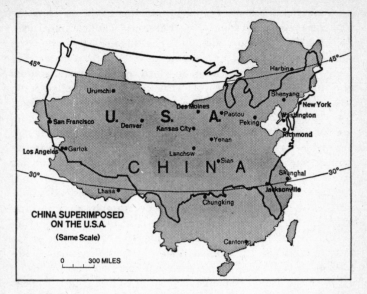

FIGURE 1. Map of China superimposed on a map of the United States. (Reprinted, with permission, from Edgar Snow, *Red China Today,* © 1970 by Random House, Inc.)

tion of southeast China which is subtropical, and northwest and northeast China which have climates closer to that of parts of Canada. More of China's land is inhospitable than is ours, however, and somewhat less of it is arable.

China's land is the home of what is by far the world's largest population. Precise figures are unknown, but estimates of the current population range from 750 to 800 million. Only India, with 585 million people, even approaches China in population (Figure 2). But in spite of China's large size it is by no means the world's most densely populated country. That dubious honor is shared by countries such as Bangladesh with a population density of 1,360 people per square mile, Japan with 750, and India with 460, all of which far exceed China's 210 (Figure 3). The population is, however, most unevenly distributed. The vast majority of the people live in eastern China, with its three great river basins;

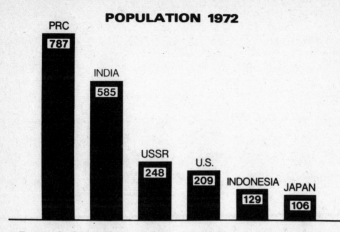

FIGURE 2. Comparison of China's population with those of other selected countries. (United Nations estimates, 1972, in millions.)

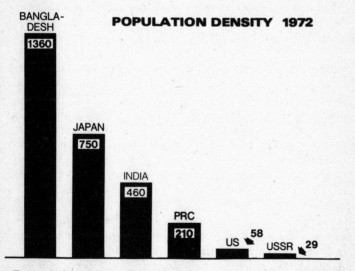

FIGURE 3. Comparison of the population density in China with those of other selected countries. (United Nations estimates, 1972, of people per square mile.)

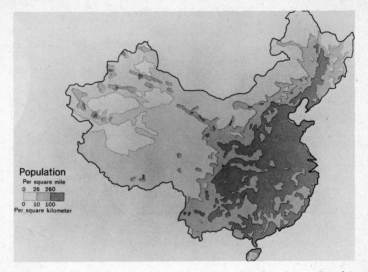

FIGURE 4. Population distribution in China. (Reprinted from *People's Republic of China Atlas,* U.S. Government Printing Office, 1971.)

western China, with its mountains and deserts, is exceedingly sparsely populated (Figure 4). The four least densely populated sections—Inner Mongolia, Sinkiang, Tsinghai, and Tibet—comprise just over half of the area of the country, but contain less than 4 per cent of the population. Both the resulting sparseness and density of population lead to problems in health care delivery. Furthermore, as will be discussed in greater detail in Chapter II, 80 per cent of the people live in rural areas, an almost exact reverse of the situation in the United States where 73 per cent of the population is urban.

Finally, we cannot emphasize strongly enough the fact that China is still a very poor country, technologically far behind not only the Western countries but Japan and the Soviet Union. Although the gross national product (GNP) per capita is an inadequate way to compare wealth among diverse societies, par-

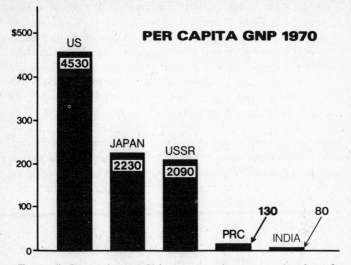

FIGURE 5. Comparison of China's per capita gross national product with those of other selected countries. (United States Government estimates, 1970, in U.S. dollars [1969].) .

ticularly among societies where the wealth is distributed in very different ways, it is a commonly used measure: China's GNP per capita is one-thirtieth that of the United States (Figure 5). More specifically, China, with almost four times as many people, produces one-thirtieth the electric power and one-seventh the crude steel produced by the United States. China has about 60,000 automobiles, a ratio of one for every 13,000 inhabitants, while the United States, with its 92 million automobiles, has slightly less than one for every two inhabitants. Conversely, China has seven commercial vehicles for every passenger vehicle, while the United States has five passenger vehicles for every commercial vehicle. The Chinese have, in fact, made the decision that automobiles will be available only for use as taxis and for official transportation, and not for private ownership. In agriculture, labor-intensive rather than mechanized methods are used and, despite the fact that China has one-fifth the amount of cultivable land per person as in United States, its output is such that not only can it now feed its own people, it has become an exporter of food.

This is not the place to discuss whether the Chinese, with their limited technological development, have a quality of life better or worse, more or less human, than ours, with our technological overdevelopment and its attendant problems. The point we make here is quite different. It is that China's health services have had to deal with the needs of a vast country and an even greater population, predominantly rural, unevenly distributed, and extremely poor compared to the technologically developed countries. How the People's Republic of China has responded to, and the ways in which it is currently attempting to meet, the medical needs of its people is the subject of this report.

I. The Development
of Health Services

THE characterization of China in the first half of this century as the "Sick Man of Asia" was largely used metaphorically. It referred to China's technological backwardness, its inability to feed its people and to provide them with other necessities of life, and its defenselessness in the face of economic and military onslaughts from the technologically developed nations. In its metaphorical sense this characterization may have been over-stated. As Bertrand Russell pointed out as early as 1922, there were strengths in the Chinese tradition and culture that were likely to enable it in time not only to provide adequately for its people but to lead them in the construction of a modern society that could match or outshine the glorious, productive, satisfying aspects of its past.[1] China's metaphorical sickness was superficial—it awaited the leadership and philosophy that could heal it.

In a literal sense, however, China's sickness was very deep and very extensive indeed. The country was plagued with almost every known form of nutritional and infectious disease. Although reliable data on incidence and prevalence are unavailable, the list of diseases caused by bacterial invaders in China included cholera, leprosy, meningococcal meningitis, plague, relapsing fever, tuberculosis, typhoid fever, and typhus. Viral illnesses included Japanese B encephalitis, smallpox, and trachoma. Diseases due to parasitic onslaughts included ancylostomiasis (hookworm), clonorchiasis, filariasis, kala-azar, malaria, paragonimiasis, and schistosomiasis.[2,3] Venereal disease was widespread. Nutritional illnesses included most known forms of total calorie, pro-

17

tein, and specific vitamin deficiencies, including beriberi, osteo-
malacia, pellagra, and scurvy; "malnutrition" was often a
euphemism for starvation.[4]

Not only are data on morbidity rates unavailable, which is not
surprising, but the few available data on mortality rates are
grossly unreliable. One estimate of the crude death rate in China
made in 1943 by Szeming Sze, secretary-general of the Chinese
Medical Association, was 25 deaths per 1,000 population annually,
more than double the rate of the technologically developed countries at that time.[5] By subtracting the death rates of Western
countries from that of China, Dr. Sze estimated that his country
had some 4 million "unnecessary" deaths each year; he attributed
75 per cent of these deaths to gastrointestinal diseases, pulmonary
tuberculosis, and infectious diseases in infants. The infant mortality rate was estimated to be 200 deaths in the first year of life per
1,000 live births. In other words, one baby in five died during its
first year.

The translation of these data into words expressing the human
misery they produced is almost impossible. Some provinces had
a folk saying: "The women conceive every year, but no child
survives to toddle along the road." [6] A Westerner who had lived in
pre-1949 Shanghai wrote in 1966 of his return to China and his
search for the sights he had known:

> I searched for scurvy-headed children. Lice-ridden children. Chil-
> dren with inflamed red eyes. Children with bleeding gums. Chil-
> dren with distended stomachs and spindly arms and legs. I searched
> the sidewalks day and night for children who had been purposely
> deformed by beggars. Beggars who would leech on to any well-
> dressed passer-by to blackmail sympathy and offerings, by pretend-
> ing the hideous-looking child was their own.
>
> I looked for children covered with horrible sores upon which
> flies feasted. I looked for children having a bowel movement,
> which, after much strain, would only eject tapeworms.
>
> I looked for child slaves in alleyway factories. Children who
> worked twelve hours a day, literally chained to small press punches.
> Children who, if they lost a finger, or worse, often were cast into
> the streets to beg and forage in garbage bins for future subsistence.[7]

One of the roots of the sickness of course was the cruel poverty
in which the vask bulk of the population lived, a poverty made

all the more cruel in the light of the wealth that had been removed from China by foreign entrepreneurs, and the relative affluence in which the small fraction of wealthy Chinese landlords and businessmen lived. Under such circumstances of poverty, medical care might have made relatively little difference in health conditions even if medical resources had been adequate. But compounding these overwhelming needs was the gross inadequacy and unavailability of health workers and medical facilities.

Health Manpower in Pre-Liberation China

The history of medical manpower in China before Liberation· is a dual one, with little interchange between the two streams.[8] It is a history, on the one hand, of traditional Chinese medical practitioners who by legend were practicing herb medicine some thirty centuries before the beginning of the Christian era; on the other hand, it is a history of the introduction from abroad of what the Chinese call "doctors of Western medicine," followed by the training of such doctors in China.

The practitioners of traditional Chinese medicine varied greatly in their training and skills, and the absence of any well-defined national qualifications for these doctors prior to Liberation makes it very difficult to estimate their number. Knud Faber, in his study for the League of Nations in 1930, was told that there were 1.2 million traditional practitioners and 7 million "druggists," but, as Croizier points out, this probably included "every kind of old-style healer and drug peddler." [9] When qualifications for doctors of Chinese medicine were formally defined by the government in 1955, the total number for the entire nation was given as 486,700.[10] It is therefore not unreasonable to estimate the number of traditional doctors in 1949 at about 500,000, or about one for every 1,100 of the estimated 540 million population at that time.

Although the definition of a doctor of Western medicine is considerably simpler, estimates of their number are almost as varied as those of traditional doctors. In 1932 there were 2,919 registered Western doctors in China, 65 per cent of whom were practicing in the three coastal provinces of Kiangsu, Kwangtung, and Chekiang.[11] In 1934 the president of the Chinese Medical

Association estimated that there were "over 6,000 scientifically-trained doctors in China." [12]

In 1943, in the midst of the war with Japan, Dr. Sze estimated that there were 12,000 doctors of Western medicine in China, of whom he stated that:

> (a) only 60 per cent of the total are duly qualified doctors, the balance being apprentice-trained practitioners who were permitted to register up to 1937; (b) 75 per cent are concentrated in the main ports of the six coastal provinces; (c) 92 per cent are under the age of 50, and 67 per cent under the age of 40, showing the relatively recent development of medical schools. [13]

Chinese estimates of the number of doctors of Western medicine at the time of Liberation vary from 20,000 to 41,400, [14] while some Western estimates are as low as 10,000 [15] or 12,000. [16] Thus the Western doctor-population ratio in 1949 may have been as low as 1:50,000 or as "high" as 1:13,000. The United States at that time had a ratio of 1:750 [17]—China would have needed some 700,000 doctors in 1949 to match that ratio.

During the years prior to 1949, attempts had been made to increase the number of Western-type health personnel, but the major effort had been devoted to training physicians following European or American models. Some observers called for new types of health personnel and new forms of training—notable among these were Faber, whose report called for "special medical schools" to increase the number of graduating physicians to 5,000 a year, [18] compared to the fewer than 200 that were graduated annually up to 1929, and John Grant, who described "medical-helpers" working through rural health stations [19]—but relatively little came of these suggestions. Even under the pressure of the war against Japan, and the concomitant aid from the United States, the "Emergency Medical Services Training Schools" that were set up did little to meet the estimated need for some 30,000 medical officers. [20]

Hospital facilities in which medical manpower might practice were similarly limited. Sze estimated that there were 38,000 hospital beds in all of China in 1943. [21] The range of estimates of the number of hospital beds in 1949 is wide; a recent one given by Chinese physicians visiting Canada in 1971 was 90,000.[22] To match the 1949 United States ratio of beds to population, China would have needed roughly 5 million beds. Even worse, these minimal resources for "scientific medicine" were concentrated, as were the doctors, in the cities.

In short, the only medical care available to the vast bulk of China's population in the rural areas, and to the majority of the poor urban population, was that provided by traditional practitioners and herbalists, many of them inadequately trained even in traditional Chinese medicine. Preventive medicine was almost nonexistent, and the cycle of poverty, disease, and disability seemed to many to be endless and immutable.

MEDICINE FROM LIBERATION TO CULTURAL REVOLUTION

It therefore comes as no surprise that a pragmatic revolutionary like Mao Tse-tung should as early as the 1930s have placed health care high on the priority list of his Chinese Communist Party and People's Liberation Army. As each village was wrested —the word our Chinese hosts use with pride is "liberated"—from the control of the Kuomintang or the Japanese, the first objectives of the liberating forces included land reform, mobilization of the peasants, and health care. These priorities are commemorated in many current Chinese art forms—written, painted, sung, acted, and danced—showing army medical personnel ministering to the peasants. We observed kindergarten children in Peking being told the story of Norman Bethune in which an important element was his service not only to wounded soldiers but to sick and injured civilians.

With Liberation—the assumption of state power by the Chinese Communist Party in 1949—health care retained its high priority and visibility. A combination of directives from Chairman Mao and principles adopted at a National Health Congress in Peking in the early 1950s resulted in a set of precepts which to this day form the widely quoted ideologic basis for the development of health services.

1. Medicine must serve the working people—in the Chinese idiom, *gong-nong-bing,* "workers, peasants, and soldiers."

2. Preventive medicine must be given priority over curative medicine.

3. Practitioners of Chinese traditional medicine (*zhongyi*) must be "united" with practitioners of Western medicine (*xiyi*).

4. Health work must be integrated with mass movements.

Implementation of these principles in the 1950s was in large measure influenced, and in part diverted, by the rapid influx of consultants, technology, and methods of organization from the Soviet Union. Medical education was largely remolded around the Soviet system of separate "faculties" for adult medicine, pediatrics, public health, stomatology, and pharmaceutics, with students differentiated early into the separate streams. Developing poly-clinics followed Soviet organizational models, with separate de-partments, for example, of medicine, surgery, and obstetrics-gynecology. Also adopted was the Soviet system of incentive rewards, ranging from membership in the prestigious Academy of Medical Sciences to considerably higher pay for professors and chiefs. Even preventive medicine, in a society with vastly different disease problems and different cultural and societal characteris-tics, followed the Soviet organizational model of "sanepid" (sanitation-epidemiology) stations, separated organizationally, con-ceptually, and attitudinally from the medical care components of the system. Categories of medical personnel ranged from "assistant doctors" (following the model of the Soviet feldsher) and nurses trained for three years in "middle" or "secondary" medical schools following completion of junior high school, to highly specialized doctors trained at the site of the Peking Union Medical College, which was reopened as an eight-year school, the China Medical College, in the late 1950s. A superb review and analysis of China's health services in the 1950s was written in 1957 by a skilled Western observer, Theodore F. Fox, editor of *The Lancet*, on the basis of a visit to China by a British medical group. Fox recog-nized what he called the "victories on many fronts," but was critical of many aspects of the system.[23]

Yet over a period of only fifteen years—from 1950 to 1965—

changes were accomplished in the delivery of health services to, and in the health of, 600 million people—an achievement apparently unprecedented in extent and rapidity in the history of the world. Cholera, plague, smallpox, and most nutritional illnesses quickly disappeared; opium addiction was eliminated, largely through community-based efforts; [24] venereal disease took somewhat longer, but by a combination of social and medical techniques was reportedly almost completely wiped out in most of China by the early 1960s.[25] Through the Great Patriotic Health Movements, the people were mobilized against the "four pests" (at first, flies, mosquitos, rats, and sparrows, with the sparrows later being replaced in the list of public enemies by bedbugs). As the process was described in 1971, "old customs and habits of the people were changed," "society was remolded," and "a new social attitude of 'regarding hygiene as an honor' took root among the mass of our people." [26]

Health care personnel were trained at an astonishing rate. Although data on the total number of medical care personnel vary, some official figures were issued for the years 1949 to 1958; in 1957 Fox was given the estimate of 70,000 doctors.[27] Since then, data have been less easily available. Those that could be found from 1958 to 1968 have been gathered and cogently integrated and analyzed by Orleans,[28] who estimates that at the end of 1966 there were about 150,000 doctors of Western medicine in China—an increase of over 100,000 doctors in less than twenty years! Other estimates, however, cite much higher and lower figures.* If we take Orleans's figure and assume a 1966 population of 725 million, the ratio of 1:5,000 would still be grossly inadequate judged by Western standards of medical care needs.

Furthermore, these doctors were still concentrated in the

* To illustrate the wide range of current estimates of the number of Western-type physicians in China, the dean of the Faculty of Medicine of the University of New South Wales in Australia in 1970 cited one doctor per 22,000 inhabitants (approximately 35,000 doctors),[29] unquestionably too low. In correspondence, he cites as his source Dean Danaraj of the Faculty of Medicine of the University of Malaya, whose February 1963 figures were in turn said to be derived from World Health Organization statistics. Croizier gives a 1966 estimate of "approximately 200,000 fully trained modern physicians (five-year medical college graduates).[30] The point is of course that truly reliable figures are as yet unavailable.

cities, although efforts were being made to shift this new manpower into the countryside; the Ministry of Health reported in
1965 that "most of 1963's 25,000 graduate doctors were channeled
into county hospitals and mining enterprises." [31]

Another major source of medical manpower, again following
the Soviet model, was the development of "secondary medical
schools." One estimate is that there were 170 such schools in
1957, 200 in 1964, and 230 in 1965.[32] In the autonomous region
of Sinkiang, for example, which is China's most western and
therefore most isolated region, there were said to be only eighteen
doctors prior to Liberation. Since 1949 a medical college and
six secondary medical schools have been built in Sinkiang.[33]

Large numbers of assistant doctors, nurses, midwives, pharmacists, and radiology and laboratory technicians have been trained
in China's secondary medical schools. The description of these
schools bears a startling resemblance to the Soviet "secondary"
or "middle" schools that train similar types of personnel as well
as "dentists." Orleans estimates that at the end of 1966 there
were in China approximately 172,000 assistant doctors, 186,000
nurses, 42,000 midwives, and 100,000 pharmacists.[34] Furthermore,
forerunners of what during the Cultural Revolution were to
become known as "barefoot doctors" were trained in the late
1950s and early 1960s in the rural areas surrounding Shanghai.[35]

In addition, Orleans estimates that among the graduates of
"higher medical education," of which physicians were the most
numerous, there were at the end of 1966 some 30,000 dentists,
whom the Soviets would at this level of training call stomatologists,
and 20,000 pharmacists, or "pharmacologists," to distinguish
them from the middle medical school pharmacy graduates, who
might be called "dispensers."

Great efforts were made during the period from Liberation to
the Cultural Revolution to integrate doctors of traditional Chinese medicine with doctors of Western medicine and to make
better use of the former. This movement began in the early
1950s with the directive by Chairman Mao that Western medicine
was to be combined as much as possible with Chinese medicine.
But despite these efforts, the marriage, described in detail by
Croizier,[36] was apparently a shaky one.

It appears that the training of doctors of Chinese medicine during this period was by both apprenticeship and formal school methods. In 1966 there were said to be twenty-one Chinese medical colleges with a total of over 10,000 students. Orleans estimates that about 1,000 doctors of Chinese medicine and 5,000 apprentices, or assistants to them, were graduated annually from 1949 to 1965.[37] It is difficult to know how to combine the figures on these graduates, who may have numbered as many as 100,000 during the seventeen years from 1949 to 1965, with the estimate of 500,000 traditional Chinese doctors at the start of the period. The closest estimate that can be made at present is to assume that the new graduates did little more than replace those who retired or died, leaving the total at about 500,000 in 1965.

Overall, then, Table 1 would appear to constitute a reasonably informed estimate of medical manpower in China at the time the Cultural Revolution began in 1966, based on limited Chinese

TABLE 1. ESTIMATED NUMBER OF MEDICAL PERSONNEL IN THE
PEOPLE'S REPUBLIC OF CHINA, 1966

| | | Ratios * | |
Type of Personnel	Number	Health Workers: 100,000 Population	Population: Health Worker
Graduates of schools of "Western" medicine			
"Higher-level" schools			
Doctors	150,000	21	4,800
Stomatologists	30,000	4	24,000
Pharmacists	20,000	3	36,000
"Middle-level" schools			
Assistant doctors	170,000	23	4,300
Nurses	185,000	26	3,900
Midwives	40,000	6	18,000
Dispensers	100,000	14	7,300
Practitioners of "Chinese medicine"	500,000	69	1,500

* Based on an estimated population of 725 million.

sources as interpreted by Western observers. These ratios were still low compared to Western or Soviet ratios, but represented an extraordinary increase in fifteen years.

Health facilities had been constructed with equally amazing rapidity. F. Avery Jones, another member of the 1957 British medical delegation, reported that "between 1949 and 1957, 860 new hospitals were built, averaging 350 beds." [38] This works out to one new hospital completed somewhere in China every three-and-a-half days—a total of some 300,000 beds in eight years. The Chinese physicians visiting Canada in 1971 stated that from 1949 to 1965 "the number of hospital beds was increased eight-fold," [39] implying that some 400,000 additional beds were built in the eight years from 1957 to 1965. By June 1965 a Ministry of Health official could proudly state that every county in China had at least one hospital. [40]

While technology was still grossly underdeveloped compared to that of Western countries, Japan, or the U.S.S.R., it was expanding rapidly and from all evidence the newly organized pharmaceutical industries far surpassed their troubled Soviet counterparts. There were reports of success in special areas of technological medicine such as the replantation of severed limbs and the salvage of patients with extensive burns. [41-47] Even here the importance of teamwork by health workers and the mobilization of the patient in the "struggle" against his illness were emphasized. Basic research was limited, but appeared to be active and successful in the laboratories of the Chinese Academy of Sciences (Academia Sinica) and of the Chinese Academy of Medical Sciences. The total synthesis of biologically-active insulin by the Biochemical Institute of the Academy of Sciences in 1965 was an example of the accomplishments. [48] Considerable clinical research was also being done, particularly under the auspices of the Academy of Medical Sciences. The contents page of the January 1963 issue of the *Chinese Medical Journal* shows some of the range of projects and the sites where research was undertaken (Figure 6). Overall, by the mid-1960s there seemed to have developed a socially-oriented, prevention-oriented, and reasonably well-rounded health care system, that had a long way to go to

中華醫學雜誌外文版

CHINESE MEDICAL JOURNAL

| Vol. 82, No. 1 | OFFICIAL ORGAN OF THE
CHINESE MEDICAL ASSOCIATION | January, 1963 |

CONTENTS

CHINESE MEDICAL ASSOCIATION
CHU SHIH TA CHIEH, PEKING, CHINA

Published by the **PEOPLE'S MEDICAL PUBLISHERS,**   Peking, China

FIGURE 6. Table of contents of the *Chinese Medical Journal,* January 1963.

meet China's needs, but that had made enormous progress in the distribution and quality of its services and in the health of the population it served.

IMPACT OF THE CULTURAL REVOLUTION

In short, it appeared to outside observers—and seemed to have appeared to many Chinese leaders at the time—that the Ministry of Health had done the job assigned to its reasonably well considering the point from which it started and the paucity of its resources in relation to the job to be done. Yet in 1965 the ministry was considered by Mao and the many others who followed his "mass line" to have failed to accomplish its goals in several key areas.

1. Despite recognition of the importance of distributing additional resources to the rural areas, and some success in doing so, urban health services still received a disproportionately large share of the limited resources. With 80 per cent of the population living in the countryside, the disproportion was a glaring one.

2. Despite recognition of the importance of preventive medicine and the striking success of a number of programs, curative medicine still received more attention in research, teaching, and service than did preventive medicine.

3. Despite recognition of the importance of integrating traditional Chinese medicine with Western medicine and some limited success at doing so, traditional medicine still received relatively short shrift and low status compared to "scientific" medicine.

4. Despite recognition of the importance of modifying techniques borrowed from other countries to fit China's unique conditions, rather than adopting them uncritically, much of medical education, public health, and medical care administration introduced into China from 1949 to the early 1960s was copied directly from Soviet models.

5. Despite recognition of the importance of collective leadership and the use of education and persuasion rather than "commandism" to implement policies, a hierarchical managerial struc-

ture developed, the top of which was said to be relatively unresponsive to criticisms or suggestions from the bottom.

6. Despite recognition of the importance of speedily assuring that everyone in the society had access to the limited medical resources, there was increasing concern with "raising of standards" rather than with "popularization" of what was already available. It was said, for example, that the force of barefoot-doctor-type health workers that had been organized near Shanghai was decreased in the name of "quality." [49]

7. Finally, and perhaps most important of all in the eyes of Mao and his associates, despite recognition of the importance of managers keeping in touch with those they served—and of breaking with the tradition of intellectual work being valued more highly than manual work—these key Maoist principles appeared to be honored more in the breach than in the observance.

Mao singled out the Ministry of Health for criticism in a statement made on June 26, 1965. Although the statement was reprinted as a *Red Medical Battle Bulletin* during the Cultural Revolution,[50] to our knowledge it has never been published in its entirety as an "official" document in any of the formal policy organs such as *Renmin Ribao* (*People's Daily*) or *Hong Chi* (*Red Flag*), or even in the *Chinese Medical Journal* or *China's Medicine*. Nonetheless, Mao's comments that "the Health Ministry renders service to only 15 per cent of the nation's population," and that it "should better be renamed the Urban Health Ministry or the 'Lords'' Health Ministry" became well known in China. The final sentence of the statement—"In medical and health work, put the stress on the rural areas!"—was widely published, became known as the "June 26th Directive," and was still quoted to us several times each day during our 1971 visit. In his statement Mao presented several prescriptions for action:

—On Medical Education: Three years in medical school after primary school are enough: "the more books you read, the more stupid you become"; after completion of medical school the students should continue the "improvement of their skill through unceasing practice."

—On Medical Research: Less men and materials should be devoted to the "peak" problems—the highly complex and hard-to-cure diseases—and more should be devoted to "the prevention and improved treatment of common diseases . . . the masses' greatest needs."

—On Medical Service: All doctors, except those who "are not extremely proficient," should "go to the rural villages" to practice.

Official statement or not, those who took charge of health care institutions during the Cultural Revolution, which began in 1966, made every effort to follow the "line" set forth by Mao and to reject what was called the "counterrevolutionary line" of the "renegade, scab, and hidden traitor," Liu Shao-ch'i, who had been Mao's successor as chairman of the People's Republic of China. The Ministry of Health and the Chinese Medical Association were particular targets of the "struggle, criticism, and transformation" of the Cultural Revolution. In October 1966 the *Chinese Medical Journal* was replaced by *China's Medicine,* a frankly political and polemical journal.

A "To Our Readers" statement in an early issue of *China's Medicine* epitomizes the rhetoric as well as the priorities of the period from late 1966 to roughly 1971:

> The Great Proletarian Cultural Revolution, unprecedented in history, which was initiated and has been led by our most respected and beloved great teacher, great leader, great supreme commander and great helmsman, Chairman Mao Tse-tung himself, constitutes a new, deeper and more extensive stage in the development of our country's socialist revolution. Our people are out to eradicate all the old ideas, old culture, old customs and old habits of the exploiting classes and foster the new ideas, new culture, new customs and new habits of the proletariat. The whole face of society and the mental outlook of the masses of the people have undergone a great transformation.

> In the course of the Great Proletarian Cultural Revolution, our medical workers, under the guidance of the invincible thought of Mao Tse-tung, have been active in revolutionizing their minds, destroying the "four olds" and establishing the "four news," giving wholehearted service to the people and making further contributions to the progress of medicine. . . We will hold still higher the great red banner of Mao Tse-tung's thought, creatively study and apply Chairman Mao's works and continuously advance

the revolutionization of our ideology and work, so that we may better serve the Chinese people and the revolutionary people of the world.[51]

The contents page of *China's Medicine* for January 1968 (five years after the contents shown in Figure 6) is reproduced in Figure 7. It demonstrates better than any summary the government's chief concerns at the height of the Cultural Revolution. Even so, *China's Medicine* ceased publication at the end of 1968.

During the Cultural Revolution medical schools admitted no new classes; students already in school were given accelerated programs of practical training and assigned to work in the countryside. Medical school faculty members, researchers in the institutes of the Academy of Medical Sciences, and other urban health workers spent periods in the rural areas performing manual labor and carrying out medical work such as training barefoot doctors, providing consultation and continuing education for medical workers, offering direct medical and preventive services, and mobilizing the peasants to play a major role in their own health care. Today, urban personnel continue to be assigned to the countryside—either to specific locations, such as a commune or county hospital, or on "mobile medical teams." As many as one-third of the staff of an urban hospital may be away at any given time—they spend six months to a year in the rural areas, and may return to visit their families twice during a year's rotation. If they choose to spend longer than a year in the countryside, they may take their families with them; a number of urban doctors are said to have relocated "permanently."

Another important reason given for the rustification was the "reeducation" of urban doctors, teachers, and researchers through hard work and contact with peasants. Those who had been through this told us in 1971 and 1972 of their changes in attitude. They described their previously inadequate appreciation of the exceedingly hard life of the peasant, and described how with a sharpened understanding of the peasant's needs came an increased dedication to service. The period of "reeducation" and the arduousness of the experience apparently was dependent on the previous "record" and "attitude" of the medical person-

CHINA'S MEDICINE

Official Organ of the
Chinese Medical Association

Number 1   January 1968

CONTENTS

FIGURE 7.   January 1968 table of contents of *China's Medicine,*
which replaced the *Chinese Medical Journal* in 1966. It was published
through December 1968.

nel, and on the nature of their responses to the experience. Despite tales of what appeared to the Western visitor as very harassing and difficult times, those telling the stories invariably ended them by recounting the ways in which their subsequent work had been improved by the experience.

Although there were precedents for the development of what in the West would be called "auxiliaries" prior to 1965, and even prior to 1949, the Cultural Revolution brought a rapid addition of new forms of health manpower very different from the regular doctors and the secondary medical personnel. These new types of health workers are not counted in the statistics as medical workers. They are counted as, and apparently consider themselves to be, primarily agricultural workers (barefoot doctors), production workers (worker doctors), or housewives and retired people (Red Medical Workers).

Further great changes have taken place in the organization of medical care—and of all institutions in Chinese society—in the wake of the Cultural Revolution. One of the issues underlying this upheaval was said to be the development since 1949 of a managerial and intellectual elite—a counterrevolutionary trend in the view of Mao and his supporters and of the substantial group to his left. Yet another issue, discussed largely by analysts outside China, was a dispute over the relative roles of the Communist Party, the army, and other groups in determining policy. During the Cultural Revolution, the direction and leadership of every organization or "unit," and in some cases the function and even the existence of the unit, was reexamined.

By the fall of 1971 the administrative leadership of all important institutions, including those dealing with health, was in the hands of "revolutionary committees" chosen on the basis of a "three-in-one" combination: one or more representatives of the People's Liberation Army, one or more cadre* members, and representatives of the "mass" who, in the case of medical care

* "Cadre" is a word used to denote "anyone in a responsible position in any organization of government, party, industry, agriculture, military, or cultural life; a key word in Chinese Communist terminology, cadre also implies ideal leadership and loyalty," but not necessarily membership in the Chinese Communist Party.[52]

institutions, are professional doctors, nurses, and other health workers. One member of the committee is selected, by processes that apparently vary from institution to institution, as the "leading" or "responsible" member. The word "chairman" is seldom used, we were told, because it implies a permanence of position that is neither intended nor desired. Anyone in a factory, a commune, or a hospital, it was emphasized, might be chosen for such a position. By 1972 the revolutionary committees seemed to have lost some of their power, and the role of professionals seemed somewhat on the ascendency.

Another extremely important leadership element, whose relationship to the revolutionary committees was not made completely clear to us and may indeed vary from institution to institution, is that of the Communist Party. We were told in 1971 that the party had 17 million members (official 1973 data stated 28 million) organized into branches in every major institution. The party branch and its leader, the branch secretary, seem to have important roles in seeing that each institution's policy is consistent with overall national and local policies. But the party role at the time of our visits appeared to be one of working closely with revolutionary committees and workers in setting policy—which the revolutionary committees then implement—rather than in making policy by decree.

Finally, the Cultural Revolution led to the reduction of salary, status, and role differences among medical personnel with different levels of expertise. Prior to the Cultural Revolution, following the Soviet model significant salary differentials had started to develop among medical care personnel and between senior medical personnel and other people in the society. Doctors who were very senior in specialization or in academic status sometimes earned four to five times as much as a beginning doctor or a factory worker. One of the results of the revolution was the decision that salaries at the upper end of the range should be frozen until salaries at the lower end rose to meet them. There was no attempt to reduce salaries, we were told, because "once people have learned to live at a certain standard it is very hard to reduce it."

With regard to status and role, changes were attempted. Efforts had already been made prior to 1965 to improve interaction among health workers. These efforts have been intensified since the Cultural Revolution. In Hangchow, for example, we were told that a pharmacist was now the "responsible member" of a district hospital. Nurses, we were told, play an important role in medical decision making, and doctors—on principle—perform tasks often "relegated" in other countries to nurses or other health workers. The object, our hosts stated, was to break down the hierarchical structure that persisted in health care institutions and to provide a setting in which all the personnel can work together more effectively for the benefit of the patients.

By the time of our visit in September-October 1971 some medical schools had admitted their first experimental post-Cultural Revolution classes—but with markedly shortened curricula and with emphasis on the practical rather than on the theoretical. Medical students were being chosen not so much on academic criteria—which had led, we were told, to the perpetuation of an intellectual elite—as on the recommendations of fellow workers or peasants based on criteria of attitude and ideology. A past record of devoted service—often in a health work role such as that of the barefoot doctor—seemed a common characteristic of the students we met.

During our 1971 visit we found that research also had markedly shifted in its orientation. "Basic" research was sharply curtailed and goal-oriented research, particularly on "common diseases" such as bronchitis, was the order of the day. Much research effort was also newly devoted to traditional Chinese medical techniques such as acupuncture, including its experimental use as an analgesic during major surgery, and the use of traditional herbs.

During our 1971 visit all attempts to meet with officials of the Ministry of Health were denied with the explanation that the ministry was still undergoing "struggle, criticism, and transformation." Our efforts to gather data for any administrative unit larger than an individual commune, factory, neighborhood, or school were also denied on the grounds that the disruptions of

中华医学杂志
CHINESE MEDICAL JOURNAL   No. 1   Jan. 1973

ABSTRACTS OF ARTICLES

FIGURE 8. Table of contents of the *Chinese Medical Journal*, which resumed publication in January 1973.

the Cultural Revolution made this impossible. Mao buttons, red-covered booklets of Mao's quotations (with an introduction by Lin Piao, whose disappearance from public view coincided with our first visit), and statues and posters of Mao were everywhere.

By the time of our second visit, in September-October 1972, much had apparently changed. Much of the visible evidence of Mao had disappeared except for the formal portraits in classrooms, conference rooms, and in people's homes; the red-covered book of quotations was less in evidence and those we saw were copies of a new edition that omitted the Lin introduction. But most important of all in our understanding of current health services in China, the "far leftward" swing of the pendulum during the Cultural Revolution seemed to have been reversed. This was seen in areas of service, education, and research, and is exemplified by the appointment in 1973 of the first minister of health since 1967 (see Chapter VIII), and by the reappearance of a *Chinese Medical Journal* devoid of political material. In Chinese, with abstracts in English, the table of contents of the first issue (Figure 8) may usefully be compared with the contents of issues five and ten years previously (Figures 6 and 7). Where, and indeed whether, the pendulum will pause in its swing is not yet clear.

NOTES

1. Bertrand Russell, *The Problem of China* (London: George Allen and Unwin, 1922).

2. James S. Simmons et al., *Global Epidemiology*, vol. 1, pt. 2 (Philadelphia: Lippincott, 1944): pp. 34-76.

3. Huang Kun-yen, "Infectious and Parasitic Diseases," in *Medicine and Public Health in the People's Republic of China*, ed. Joseph R. Quinn (Washington, D.C.: National Institutes of Health, 1972): pp. 263-88.

4. Samuel D.J. Yeh and Bacon F. Chow, "Nutrition," in Quinn, Ibid., pp. 211-38.

5. Szeming Sze, *China's Health Problems* (Washington, D.C.: Chinese Medical Association, 1943).

6. *For the Health of the People* (Peking: Foreign Languages Press, 1963).

7. W. A. Scott, "China Revisited by an Old China Hand," *Eastern Horizon* 5, no. 6 (June, 1966): 34-40.

8. Ralph C. Croizier, *Traditional Medicine in Modern China* (Cambridge: Harvard University Press, 1968): p. 37.

9. Knud Faber, *Report on Medical Schools in China* (Geneva: League of Nations, Health Organization, 1931), cited in Croizier, Ibid., n. 21, pp. 265-66.

10. *Jen-min Shou-ts'e (People's Handbook)* (Peking: 1957): p. 608, cited in Leo Orleans, "Medical Education and Manpower in Communist China," *Aspects of Chinese Education*, ed. C.T. Hu (New York: Teachers College Press, Columbia University, 1969): p. 31.

11. Nei-cheng Pu (Ministry of the Interior), *Ch'uan-kuo teng-chi i-shih ming-lu* (*National Register of Physicians*) (Nanking: 1933), cited in Croizier, *Traditional Medicine in Modern China*, n. 41, p. 250.

12. Way Sung New, "Some Outstanding Features of Our Work," *Chinese Medical Journal* 48 (1934): 385-91.

13. Sze, *China's Health Problems*, p. 18.

14. Orleans, "Medical Education and Manpower," p. 21.

15. Croizier, *Traditional Medicine in Modern China*, p. 157.

16. William Y. Chen, "Medicine and Public Health," in *Sciences in Communist China,* ed. Sidney Gould (Washington: 1961): p. 384, cited in Croizier, *Traditional Medicine in Modern China*, n. 20, p. 265.

17. United States Bureau of the Census, *The United States, Colonial Times to 1957* (Washington, D.C.: 1960): p. 34.

18. Faber, *Report on Medical Schools*, cited in Croizier, *Traditional Medicine in Modern China*, n. 43, p. 250.

19. John B. Grant, "Rural Reconstruction in China, in *Health Care for the Community: Selected Papers of Dr. John B. Grant*, ed. Conrad Seipp (Baltimore: The Johns Hopkins Press, 1963): pp. 148-54.

20. Croizier, *Traditional Medicine in Modern China*, p. 55.

21. Sze, *China's Health Problems*, p. 12.

22. Chen Wen-chieh and Ha Hsien-wen, "Medical and Health Work in New China." (Unpublished talk given by two Chinese physicians during a visit to Canada in November 1971).

23. Theodore F. Fox, "The New China: Some Medical Impressions," *The Lancet* 2 (November 1957): 935-39, 995-99, 1053-57.

24. Paul Lowinger, "The Politics of Drugs," *Social Policy* 3, no. 2 (July-August 1972): 41-43.

25. Ma Hai-teh, "With Mao Tse-tung's Thought as the Compass for Action in the Control of Venereal Diseases in China," *China's Medicine* no. 1 (October 1966): 52-68.

26. Chen and Ha, "Medical and Health Work."

27. Fox, "The New China."

28. Orleans, "Medical Education and Manpower," pp. 27-28.

29. F. F. Rundle, "Community Distribution of Doctors as a Challenge to Medical Education and Training," *Medical Journal of Australia* 1 (1970): 1064-65.

30. Croizier, *Traditional Medicine in Modern China*, p. 193.

31. Chang Tze-k'uan, "The Development of Hospital Services in China," *Chinese Medical Journal* 84 (1965): 412-16.

32. Orleans, "Medical Education and Manpower," p. 34.

33. "News and Notes: Medical Careers for Women of National Minorities in Sinkiang," *Chinese Medical Journal* 82 (1963): 261.

34. Orleans, "Medical Education and Manpower," p. 37.

35. "The Orientation of the Revolution in Medical Education as Seen in the Growth of 'Barefoot Doctors'," *China's Medicine* no. 10 (October 1968): 574-81.

36. Croizier, *Traditional Medicine in Modern China*, pp. 157-88.

37. Orleans, "Medical Education and Manpower," pp. 32-33.

38. F. Avery Jones, "A Visit to China," *British Medical Journal* 2 (November 1957): 1105-1107.

39. Chen and Ha, "Medical and Health Work."

40. Chang, "The Development of Hospital Services."

41. Ch'en Chung-wei, Ch'ien Yun-ch'ing, and Pao Yueh-se, "Salvage of the Forearm Following Complete Amputation." *Chinese Medical Journal* 82 (1963): 632-38.

42. Ch'en Chung-wei et al., "Further Experience in the Restoration of Amputated Limbs," *Chinese Medical Journal* 84 (1965): 225-31.

43. Huang Ch'eng-ta, Li Ping-heng, and Kong Gung-to, "Successful Restoration of a Traumatic Amputated Leg," *Chinese Medical Journal* 84 (1965): 641-45.

44. Ts'ui Chih-yi et al., "Successful Restoration of a Completely Amputated Arm," *Chinese Medical Journal* 85 (1966): 536-41.

45. Committee of the Chinese Communist Party of the Shanghai Second Medical College, "The Fight to Save Steel Worker Ch'iu Ts'ai K'ang's Life," *Chinese Medical Journal* 77 (November 1958): 414.

46. Burns Ward of the Department of Traumatology and Orthopedics, Peking Chishueit'an Hospital, "Utilize Mao Tse-tung's Thinking to the Full in Treating Burned Patients," *Chinese Medical Journal* 84 (1965): 707-13.

47. Wu Ying-k'ai, "Progress of Surgery in China," *Chinese Medical Journal* 84 (1965): 351-61.

48. Ethan Signer and Arthur W. Galston, "Education and Science in China" *Science* 175 (1972): 15-23.

49. "The Orientation of the Revolution."

50. Mao Tse-tung, "June 26 'Directive' (June 26, 1965)," *Red Medical Battle Bulletin and August 18 Battle Bulletin Commemorative Issue* (June 26, 1967), trans. in *Survey of China Mainland Press* 198 suppl. (1967):30.

51. "To Our Readers," *China's Medicine* no. 1 (January 1967): 74.

52. Edgar Snow, "Population Care and Control," *Population and Family Planning in the People's Republic of China* (Washington: Victor-Bostrom Fund Committee and Population Crisis Committee, 1971): p. 8.

II. Health Care
in the Cities

CHINA is divided into twenty-two provinces (including what our Chinese hosts called the "as yet unliberated province of Taiwan"), twenty-one of which are on the mainland of Asia (Figure 9). In addition there are five autonomous regions inhabited largely by minority ethnic groups that are relatively small in size compared to the dominant Han group which comprises 90 per cent of the population.

Three cities and their supporting countryside areas have been removed from the jurisdiction of the provinces in which they are situated and placed directly under the jurisdiction of the central government as independent municipalities. The largest of these is Shanghai, with a population of about 6 million in the city proper, and about 4 million in its surrounding ten counties. The other independent municipalities are Peking, with 4 million in the city proper and 3 million in its nine surrounding counties, and Tientsin, with a population of 4 million. A list of the provinces, autonomous regions, and centrally administered cities on the mainland, and their estimated populations, is given in Table 2.

Cities are governed by revolutionary committees—formal government bodies; their health services are coordinated by the local bureau of public health, which not only has responsibility for almost all service units and almost all health care personnel in the city, but for educational institutions for nonphysician health care personnel. The scope of the bureaus is discussed in greater detail in Chapter VIII; a recent estimate of the number

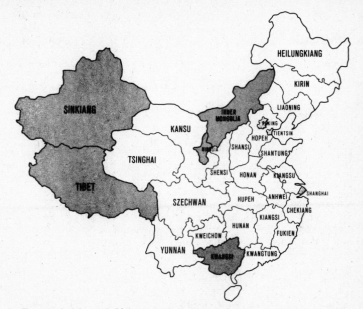

FIGURE 9. Map of China's mainland provinces, autonomous regions (Inner Mongolia, Kwangsi, Ningsia, Sinkiang, and Tibet), and independent municipalities (Peking, Shanghai, and Tientsin).

of medical workers in Peking and Shanghai is presented in Table 3.

The next lower level of urban organization is the "district," which is also governed by a revolutionary committee. Hangchow, a city of 700,000 people, is divided into four districts; the city proper of Peking into nine districts; and the city proper of Shanghai into ten districts. Districts are subdivided into "streets" or "neighborhoods," which are the lowest level of formal governmental organization in the city. The size and even the generic names of these neighborhoods vary widely through China. In Sian, for example, a unit of about 50,000 people that we visited is

TABLE 2. ADMINISTRATIVE DIVISIONS OF THE PEOPLE'S REPUBLIC
OF CHINA, 1971

Divisions	Capital	Estimated 1970 Population (in millions)
Provinces		
Anhwei	Hofei	39
Chekiang	Hangchow	31
Fukien	Foochow	18
Heilungkiang	Harbin	25
Honan	Chengchow	55
Hopei	Shihkiachwang	46
Hunan	Changsha	41
Hupei	Wuchang	35
Kansu	Lanchow	16
Kiangsi	Nanchang	25
Kiangsu	Nanking	51
Kirin	Changchun	21
Kwangtung	Kwangchow (Canton)	40
Kweichow	Kweiyang	20
Liaoning	Shenyang (Mukden)	29
Shansi	Taiyuan	20
Shantung	Tsinan	60
Shensi	Sian	22
Szechwan	Chengtu	75
Tsinghai	Sining	2.5
Yunnan	Kunming	24
Autonomous Regions		
Inner Mongolia	Huhehot	9
Kwangsi (Chuang)	Nanning	25
Ningsia (Hui)	Yinchwan	2.5
Sinkiang (Uigur)	Urumchi	10
Tibet	Lhasa	1.5
Centrally Administered Cities		
Peking		7 *
Shanghai		10 *
Tientsin		4
Estimated Total		765

Source: The "post office" spellings of the Chinese names and the estimated population data are drawn from Theodore Shabad, *China's Changing Map* (New York: Praeger, 1972): p. 34.

* These estimates include the population of the rural areas under the jurisdiction of the central city.

TABLE 3. MEDICAL PERSONNEL IN THE PEKING AND SHANGHAI INDEPENDENT MUNICIPALITIES*

	Number	Ratios	
		Health Workers: 100,000 Population	Population: Health Worker
Shanghai (10.5 million people in ten urban districts and ten rural counties)†			
Doctors of Western medicine	10,144 (9,000)	97	1,040
Doctors of Chinese medicine	4,139 (3,500)	39	2,530
Assistant (middle-grade) doctors	4,670 (4,000)	45	2,240
Nurses	20,342 (15,000)	193	520
Technicians, pharmacists, etc.	9,812 (14,000)	94	1,070
Peking (7 million people in nine urban districts and nine rural counties)‡			
Doctors of Western medicine	10,000	140	700
Doctors of Chinese medicine	2,000	30	3,500
Assistant (middle-grade) doctors	5,000	70	1,400
Nurses	11,000	160	600
Technicians, pharmacists, etc.	8,000	110	900

* These figures do not include barefoot doctors, worker doctors, or Red Medical Workers, since they are not considered primarily health manpower; some estimates of the number and distribution of barefoot doctors are presented in Chapter III.
† Data provided by the Shanghai Bureau of Public Health in October 1972; the figures in parentheses are estimates provided by the Shanghai branch of the CMA in October 1971.
‡ Estimates provided by the CMA in September 1971.

called an "urban commune"; the name is a remnant of the experimental introduction of commune structures into China's cities as part of the Great Leap Forward of 1958. The neighborhood is governed by a committee composed of representatives of the people in the area, cadres, and, in diminishing numbers since the end of the Cultural Revolution, members of the People's Liberation Army. The committee's responsibilities include the administration of local factories, primary schools and kindergartens, a neighborhood hospital or health center, repair services, and a housing department, and the organization and supervision of "residents' " or "lane" committees.

The smallest unit in the urban areas is the "lane" (or block), with from 1,000 to 8,000 residents. Some lanes are further divided into groups—for example, the residents of a single large apartment building—headed by a group or deputy group leader. The lane is governed by a committee chosen by, and from among, the "mass" living in the lane. The committee is a "mass organization" rather than a formal governmental body and thus does not usually have the three-in-one components of the revolutionary committees; the elderly play a key role in the organization and administration of these committees. Figure 10 is a schematic representation of the levels of urban organization.

HEALTH CARE IN THE LANE AND NEIGHBORHOOD

Each of the nine districts of Peking city proper, to use it as an example, has a population of about 400,000. Among the services provided at the district level are hospitals, sanitation facilities, middle schools (roughly equivalent to our junior and senior high schools), and "prevention stations" for illnesses such as tuberculosis and mental disorders.

Within each district there are "neighborhoods" consisting of approximately 50,000 people. The West District of Peking has nine neighborhoods, of which the Fengsheng neighborhood, with a population of 53,000, is one (Figure 11). Within the Fengsheng neighborhood's jurisdiction are six factories, eight shops, ten primary schools, four kindergartens, and a neighborhood hospital.

Fengsheng is one of the older neighborhoods of Peking. It

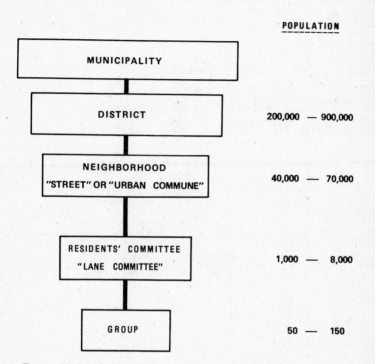

POPULATION

MUNICIPALITY

DISTRICT   200,000 — 900,000

NEIGHBORHOOD
"STREET" OR "URBAN COMMUNE"   40,000 — 70,000

RESIDENTS' COMMITTEE
"LANE COMMITTEE"   1,000 — 8,000

GROUP   50 — 150

FIGURE 10. Levels of urban organization in the People's Republic of China.

consists entirely of one-story dwellings rather than the four- or five-story apartment buildings found in newer neighborhoods. Courtyards, with several families living in each, are entered through doorways in the walls lining Fengsheng's 132 lanes. The people are grouped into twenty-five residents' committees, each of which encompasses about 2,000 people. These committees usually provide a health station and other social services. Within

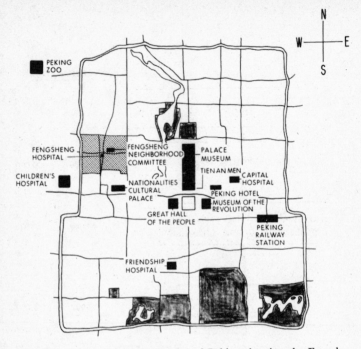

FIGURE 11. Map of the inner city of Peking showing the Fengsheng neighborhood.

each committee are organized "groups" of from fifty to 150 people led by a group leader and a deputy group leader who conduct a number of the aspects of what we might term social or welfare work.

The health workers at the residents' committee level are local housewives called "Red Medical Workers." Three such workers serve the Wu Ting residents' committee, located in the western part of the Fengsheng neighborhood. Wu Ting has 400 families totaling approximately 1,500 people. The chairman of the residents' committee, Chao Huan-ching, is a seventy-year-old retired worker. Comrade Chao also serves as the director of the Wu Ting residents' committee health station, although he is not considered a health worker.

The major function of a residents' committee health station is preventive work, although it does treat some minor illnesses. The Wu Ting station is located in a single room off one of the courtyards, and its fairly typical equipment includes a bed for examination or treatment, a table with chairs for consultations, and a cabinet containing both Western-type and traditional Chinese medicines. On the walls are a picture of Mao Tse-tung, an acupuncture chart, and health propaganda posters.

We spoke at length with two of Wu Ting's Red Medical Workers. The first, Comrade Yang Hsio-hua, is thirty-eight years of age. After her marriage she had worked briefly as a saleswoman until she was nineteen, when her first child was born. Since then she has been home taking care of her children, now aged nineteen, fifteen, and eleven. Two years ago, responding to the call to "Serve the People" which grew out of the Great Proletarian Cultural Revolution, she volunteered for one month of training in the Fengsheng neighborhood hospital. During the training period she and her fellow housewives learned history taking and simple physical examination techniques such as blood pressure determination. They were taught the uses of a number of Western and herb medicines, and techniques of acupuncture and of intra-muscular and subcutaneous injection. Preventive measures such as sanitation, immunization, and birth control procedures were an important part of the curriculum. But the most important element, we were told, was that Comrade Yang and her colleagues were taught that there are no barriers to the acquisition of medical knowledge other than their own fears. Once these are overcome, in part through sessions in which life in the "bitter past" and the feelings of the students are shared and discussed, a lifetime of continued learning is anticipated. Comrade Yang learns from the doctor at the neighborhood hospital who visits the residents' committee health station three times a week, from her own periodic visits to the hospital for instruction or to consult about a patient, and from the biweekly or monthly meetings of all the Red Medical Workers of the neighborhood.

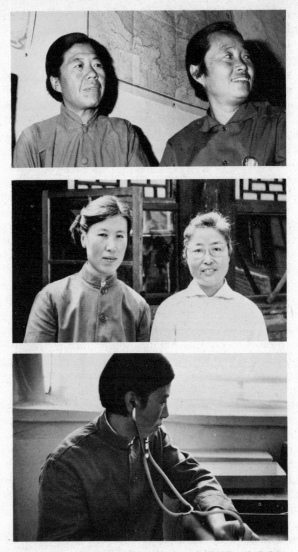

Red Medical Workers, Fengsheng neighborhood, Peking

The other Red Medical Worker with whom we talked was Chang Cheng-yu, who is forty-three years of age. Her two children are now twenty-one and twelve years old. She has been a housewife all her married life and had never worked outside the home until she became a health worker. Both Comrades Yang and Chang live in the residents' committee area within a few steps of the health station, which is staffed by them and their colleagues from 8:00 to 11:00 A.M., when they usually see from seven to ten patients, and from 3:00 to 5:30 P.M., when they see four or five more patients. If a resident feels ill when the station is closed, he or she may go directly to the home of one of the Red Medical Workers, although we were told that this rarely happens.

The health workers are paid a modest sum for their work, about 15 *yüan* a month, roughly one-third of a beginning factory worker's wages. The stipend comes in part from the small fees paid by patients, in part from the collective income of neighborhood factories and home industries. A patient's fee for a visit to the health station is never more than 10 *fen*, and usually far less. If the patient is a retired worker, he may present the health station bills to his former place of employment, where reimbursement is made in full. If the patient is a dependent of a factory worker or of one who has retired, the factory will reimburse half the health station charges. Workers currently employed are rarely seen in the health stations because their primary medical care needs are taken care of at their place of work.

A large part of the duties of the Red Medical Workers, who are supervised by the Department of Public Health of the neighborhood hospital, relates to sanitation work in the neighborhood. In the summer there are campaigns against flies and mosquitoes and attempts to prevent the spread of gastrointestinal disorders. In the winter and spring the health workers are concerned mainly with the prevention of upper respiratory infections, for which they encourage morning exercises, washing the face with cold water, long walks, the use of traditional medicines, and the use of masks when a patient has a cold to prevent its spread. The public health department also supervises the Red

Medical Workers in providing immunizations, which are usually given in the health stations.

The Red Medical Workers also have as their responsibility the provision of birth control information. They distribute oral contraceptives directly, often with no specific medical examination prior to initiation of treatment. Intrauterine contraceptive devices are available and insertion is performed by trained personnel in the neighborhood hospital. The Red Medical Workers make periodic visits to all women in the residents' committee area to encourage the use of contraception.

In addition to treating patients with minor illnesses the Red Medical Workers provide follow-up care after a patient has been treated in a hospital. For example, we saw Red Medical Workers treating patients with arthritis, using a combination of acupuncture and herb medicines. We also observed them checking blood pressures and determining the dose of medication for patients with hypertension. The therapy had been started in the neighborhood or district hospital and the continuing dose of medication prescribed. The Red Medical Worker may herself change the type of traditional medicine given to a hypertensive patient, but can only vary the dose of Western medicine within certain limits. If a patient's blood pressure is found to be outside limits set by the hospital, the patient is sent back to the hospital for treatment and new instructions.

The back-up institution for the residents' committee and factory health stations is the neighborhood hospital. In Fengsheng this hospital occupies two large courtyards and has seven departments: medicine, surgery, acupuncture, traditional bone medicine, gynecology, dentistry, and tuberculosis; and four auxiliary units: pharmacy (including both traditional Chinese and Western drugs), laboratory, X-ray, and injections. The public health department serving the neighborhood is located in the hospital, which has no beds; patients requiring hospitalization are sent to the People's Hospital in the West District, several blocks from Fengsheng.

Of the ninety staff members, twenty-seven are doctors—twenty trained in traditional Chinese medicine and seven in

Western or scientific medicine. There are thirty-one middle medical workers (nurses and technicians), eighteen administrative and other staff, and fourteen students training in the hospital following graduation from middle school. Many of those working in the hospital live in the neighborhood, although a number come from outside. Most of the doctors function as specialists, with patients assigned to them on the basis of presenting problems: a patient with a cough would go to an internist, one with an injury to a surgeon.

Salaries for hospital doctors range from 46 to 155 *yüan* per month; traditional and Western-trained doctors have the same salary scale. Nurses begin at 40 *yüan* per month; the highest-paid nurse at the hospital in the fall of 1972 earned 69 *yüan* a month. Administrative personnel earn from 40 to 70 *yüan* a month.

The director of the Fengsheng neighborhood hospital is Madame Liu Pei-pung, a short plump woman in her late forties. Before becoming director in 1970 she had been director of the Peking Women's Hospital for thirteen years. Madame Liu and Comrade Yang Lan-ying of the administrative office are the two full-time members of the all-female "leading group" or revolutionary committee of the hospital. The three others, a nurse, a pharmacist and a doctor of traditional Chinese medicine are part-time committee members. The group meets at least once a week to plan the medical work and to "study how to serve the people better." They listen to the complaints of both doctors and patients. If some doctors feel there are too many patients, the leading group organizes the doctors into study groups and helps them to change their attitudes. If a patient has a special request, such as wanting a doctor to make a home visit, the leading group tries to see that it is met.

Although the equipment in the neighborhood hospital is sparse and primitive, it seems adequate for the level of health work performed there. Simple laboratory tests and X-rays are available. The institution appears to function at a level not unlike that of many neighborhood health centers in the United States, one difference of course being the great use of traditional Chinese medical techniques. In addition, the hospital acts as a center for public health work in the neighborhood, and the coverage and intensity of this work appears to far exceed that of most such urban centers in the United States.

During the course of two hours one afternoon, Dr. Yang Yi-chin of the Department of Internal Medicine saw seventeen patients in a large room in which three other doctors were also seeing patients. The patient sat near Dr. Yang's desk while the history was taken. A simple physical examination, such as inspection of the throat or ausculation of the heart or lungs, was done with the patient sitting down. If a more complete examination was needed, the patient was taken behind a screen to the single examining table shared by all four doctors.

The results of the history taking, the examination, and the diagnosis were recorded on the left half of a form about 6-by-4 inches in size; prescriptions were written on the right side of the form. A carbon copy was made and the patient was given both copies: the original was to take to the pharmacy where it was filled and kept on file; the copy was retained by the patient, who was asked to bring it on return visits. Since the copy in the pharmacy was filed according to date rather than the name of the patient, the only unified record of care was that maintained by the patient.

Of the seventeen patients seen by Dr. Yang during the afternoon we observed him, thirteen were female and four, including a thirteen-year-old boy, were male. Six had upper respiratory infections, five high blood pressure, and the remainder a variety of other disorders amenable to ambulatory care. The following are examples of the patients Dr. Yang saw and the way they were handled:

> —A thirty-two-old woman with a history of high blood pressure complained of feeling faint and of not sleeping well. Her blood pressure was recorded as 108/178 (diastolic over systolic). Dr. Yang listened to the patient's heart under her shirt; upon examination he found slight edema in her legs. He ordered a urinalysis and the patient went to have it done in a laboratory off the hospital courtyard. She returned in approximately fifteen minutes with the results, which were normal. Dr. Yang's diagnosis was hypertension. He prescribed rauwolfia (8 mg., three times a

day, ten tablets), dibazol (20 mg., three times a day, ten tablets), perphenazine (2 mg., three times a day, ten tablets), and "librium" (chlordiazepoxide hydrochloride) (20 mg., one at bedtime, five tablets). The doctor also gave the patient a certificate excusing her from work for three days, at which time she was to return to the hospital.

—A man aged fifty-one presented slips from previous visits. He was seen two-and-a-half weeks before in the People's Hospital for a urinary tract infection; white blood cells had been found in his urine and treatment was begun. One week prior to this visit he was seen in the Fengsheng hospital by another doctor and a repeat urinalysis was done. A urinalysis had also been done just before he saw Dr. Yang. The patient complained of continued dysuria and pain in the left flank. Dr. Yang told the patient to drink more water, to continue his medicines, which consisted of kanamycin (0.5 g., twice a day, six tablets) and "furadantin" (nitrofurantoin) (0.1 g., three times a day, nine tablets), and to return in three days.

—A twenty-eight-year-old female teacher in a middle school in the neighborhood complained of mild fever for several days, weakness, lack of strength, and cough. Dr. Yang first ascertained that there was no history of tuberculosis in her family and then listened to her heart and chest, which proved to be normal. The patient told him in response to his question that her stools had been normal. Dr. Yang sent her to have a chest X-ray. The patient returned in a half-hour with the report of a normal X-ray. A laboratory test showed no increase in white blood cells. Dr. Yang prescribed "terramycin" (oxytetracycline) (0.5 g., four times a day, eight tablets) and Vitamin C (0.1 g., three times a day, twenty tablets).

In short, with some difference in treatment patterns, for example, the use of antibiotics and Vitamin C for what appeared to the observers to be a relatively mild viral upper respiratory infection, Dr. Yang's practice was similar to that of a physician in a neighborhood health center or in general practice in the United States. Outside academic centers in the United States, the difference in the way viral upper respiratory infections are treated might also be minimal.

In another Peking neighborhood adjacent to the Imperial Palace Museum we discussed the role of Red Medical Workers in the prevention of infectious diseases. (See Table 4 for the

TABLE 4. INSTRUCTIONS POSTED AT A LANE HEALTH STATION IN PEKING:
WORKING RESPONSIBILITIES OF RED MEDICAL WORKERS

---

1. Hold high the great banner of Mao Tse-tung's thought. Stand up
   for proletarian politics. Study Chairman Mao's philosophical works
   creatively. Change our world outlook. Practice and apply it in
   every day's work.
2. Strengthen revolutionary discipline. Do not be late to work, do not
   go home early, do not be "thrice divorced": divorced from the mass
   movement, divorced from physical labor, or divorced from the
   masses.
3. Stress the policy of prevention. Initiate the patriotic health movement centered around the prevention of disease. Every week there
   should be a small general cleaning and every two weeks a big general cleaning. Proceed to inspect and increase the management of
   infectious disease. Emphasize prevention and vaccination work.
   Reach the unity of prevention and treatment.
4. Work on family plannning. Do propaganda work constantly. Know
   the local situation clearly.
5. Be self-reliant. Observe the principles of diligence and frugality.
   Try to treat the patient at home. Take good care of chronic diseases. Work for the prevention of disease and the treatment of
   disease at a local level. Move forward (ride the horse of) the three
   traditions: traditional doctors, traditional medicines, and traditional methods. Use yourself creatively (collect the herbs yourself,
   make the herbs yourself, plant the herbs yourself, and use the herbs
   yourself).

"Working Responsibilities of Red Medical Workers" in one
lane health station we visited in the neighborhood.) Through
mass meetings and discussions with individual families, the Red
Medical Workers in the twenty-three lane health stations of this
neighborhood have educated the population of 49,300 about the
importance of immunizations. The Red Medical Worker also
informs parents when it is time for their children to receive
immunizations. The lane health station is very near each family's
home and therefore convenient to visit. If a family does not bring
a child to the station for immunization at the appropriate time,
however, the Red Medical Worker will sometimes bring the child
to the station, or if necessary arrange for the immunization to be

given in the home. A chart we saw in one lane health station indicated that 95 to 100 per cent of the children had been immunized against measles, diphtheria, poliomyelitis, pertussis, tetanus, encephalitis, meningitis, and tuberculosis (Table 5). Other charts for this district indicated a marked decline in recent years in the incidence of measles, poliomyelitis, diphtheria, and pertussis. About 80 per cent of the children had been vaccinated against smallpox. We were told that since the last case of smallpox in China had occurred in 1954, vaccination is not given if there is any contraindication. It is worth noting that in a society in which mass participation is an important principle, individual exceptions can be made when there is good reason to do so. "Herd immunity" tends to protect the minority who are unvaccinated, and they can be spared the risk of vaccination. Table 6 shows in detail the kinds of immunization that seem to be fairly common throughout China. The types of records kept in the lanes and in the neighborhoods are shown in Figures 12, 13, and 14.

Health workers in the lanes and neighborhoods also play an important role in birth control campaigns. In the period preceding Liberation, China's annual crude birth rate was said to be about 43 per 1,000 population.[1] After a lengthy period of widely varying policies toward population control, vigorous campaigns were launched—particularly in the cities—in the 1960s.

Education is one of the most important aspects of the program. This is done through booklets and other printed materials,

TABLE 5. CHILDHOOD IMMUNIZATION RATES AT A LANE HEALTH STATION IN PEKING, 1971

Immunization	Number Eligible	Number Immunized	Percent Immunized
Measles	160	156	97.5
Poliomyelitis	164	164	100.0
DPT	163	163	100.0
Encephalitis	119	112	94.1
Meningitis	136	132	97.0
BCG	164	163	98.1
Smallpox	163	135	80.9

TABLE 6. CHILDHOOD IMMUNIZATIONS GIVEN IN CHINA

BCG (Against tuberculosis)	Initial vaccination is performed within three days after birth. Tuberculin testing is performed every three years, and a booster BCG dose is given if the tuberculin test is negative.
Poliomyelitis	Oral (live, attenuated) vaccine is given at about six months in three doses at monthly intervals; three doses are repeated at one year, and again at age five to seven.
Triple vaccination (diptheria, pertussis, and tetanus)	The initial three doses are given at three to six months; single booster doses are given at age three and at age six.
Measles	Initial immunization is given at six to eight months to children with no history of measles; boosters are given three to five years later.
Smallpox	Initial vaccination is given at six months, with revaccination at age six. Vaccination is not given if there is any contraindication, such as exzema.
Japanese B encephalitis	Immunization is given annually in October or November to children under the age of fourteen.
Meningococcal meningitis (groups A and B)*	Immunization is given annually in October or November to children under the age of fourteen.

* The report of the apparent availability of a vaccine against meningococcus group B organisms has caused considerable interest in the United States, where polysaccharide vaccines of group A and group C *Neisseria meningitidis* are being tested and found effective, but where no effective vaccine against group B has as yet been developed. (See, for example, Editorial, "Vaccination Against Meningococcal Infection," *The Lancet* 1 [1972]: 625; and Arnold S. Monto, Brenda L. Brandt, and Malcolm S. Artenstein, "Response of Children to *Neisseria Meningitidis* Polysaccharide Vaccines," *Journal of Infectious Diseases* 127 [1973]: 394-400.) Further study will be needed to determine the nature of the difference between the vaccines developed in the two countries, and whether the report may instead be based on a linguistic misunderstanding or differences in classification of the organisms.

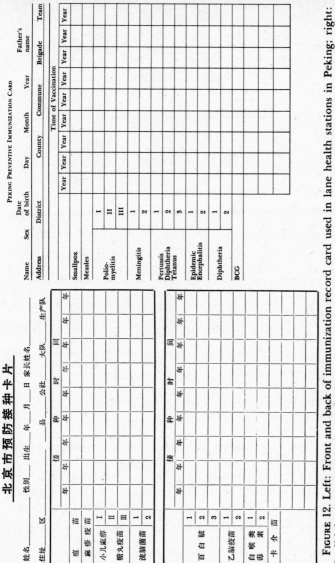

FIGURE 12. Left: Front and back of immunization record card used in lane health stations in Peking; right: English-language translation of the card.

儿 童 保 健 记 录

| 姓名： | 性别： | 出生 | 年 | 月 | 日(早产、足月、双胎)住址： |

| 家长姓名： | 工作单位： | 电话： | 经常易患何病： |

| 患过何种传染病：麻疹 年 月，水痘 年 月，腮腺炎 年 月，肝炎 年 月， |

| 百日咳 年 月 | 近月内有无接触过传染病： |

预防接种情况	项目 时间	年	年	年	年	年	年	年	项目 时间	年	年	年	年	年	年	年
	痘 苗								流脑菌苗 1 2							
	麻疹疫苗								乙脑疫苗 1 2							
	小儿麻痹疫苗 I II								白喉类毒素 1 2							
	百白破 1 2 3								卡 介 苗							

CHILDREN'S HEALTH RECORD

| Name | Sex | Date of birth | Day | Month | Year (Early birth, normal birth, twins) Address |

| Father's name | Unit of work | Tel. no. | Illnesses child has had |

| Infectious diseases child has had: Measles month year; Chicken pox month year; Mumps month year |

| Hepatitis month year; Pertussis month year | Has child been in contact with infectious diseases in recent month? |

Status of Preventive Vaccination	Item Time	Year	Year	Year	Year	Year	Year	Year	Item Time	Year	Year	Year	Year	Year	Year	Year
	Smallpox								Meningitis 1 2							
	Measles															
	Poliomyelitis I II III								Epidemic Encephalitis 1 2							
	Pertussis 1 2 3								Diphtheria 1 2							
									BCG							

FIGURE 13. Top: Front of a children's health record card used in neighborhood hospitals in Peking; bottom: English-language translation of the card.

and, even more important, through street committees, Red Medical Workers, and other person-to-person contacts. The emphasis is on the importance of family planning in building a new socialist society, rather than on the Malthusian concepts of overpopulation leading to poverty and famine. Family planning is

> based upon the emancipation of the woman, her equality, her right to study and participate in all political decisions, and her heightened social consciousness. Planned parenthood and mar-

检查日期							
实足年龄							
身长(公分)							
体重(公斤)							
营养							
前囟							
眼							
耳							
鼻							
咽喉							
牙 数							
牙 龋齿							
心							
肺							
肝							
皮肤							
佝偻病							
其他							
医生签字							

注：凡入托者注明可否入托，
正常(－)，缺点(＋、卄、卅)
早产、足月、双胎记(√)
佝偻病注明(活动期、恢复期、后遗症期或无
营养不良注明(一度、二度、三度或无)

Date of Examination						
Full Age						
Height (centimeters)						
Weight (kilograms)						
Nutrition						
Fontanelle						
Eyes						
Ears						
Nose						
Throat						
Teeth: Number						
Teeth: Caries						
Heart						
Lungs						
Liver						
Skin						
Rickets						
Other						
Signature of Doctor						

Notes: Whether child can join nursery
Normal (—)
Shortcomings (+, ++, +++)
Early birth, normal birth, twins (√)
Note the period of rickets (active, recovering, sequela, or no rickets)
Note the degree of malnutrition (first, second, third, or normal)

FIGURE 14. Left: Back of a children's health record card shown in Figure 13; right: English-language translation of the card.

riage are factors for the promotion of a socialist society, but they must be based on full equality of both partners, self-respect, and knowledge. It is therefore essential that the masses themselves should grasp all the factors of health work, and themselves carry out the programs.[2]

The Chinese marriage law of 1950 provides that women may marry at age eighteen and men at age twenty, but a vigorous and successful campaign has been waged to delay the age of marriage. In the cities the usual age for marriage for men is now said to be twenty-six to twenty-nine, and for women twenty-four to twenty-six. Late marriage is of course itself a powerful method of population control. Many first babies are being delivered to mothers in their late twenties or early thirties. The optimal family size in the cities is now considered to be two to three children, and tubal or vas deferens ligation, we were told, is often urged after the second or third child.

In the urban lanes, Red Medical Workers are responsible for the dissemination of birth control information. In Silvery Lane in Hangchow, health workers trained by Red Medical Workers from the street hospital go from door to door talking with the women about the number of children they want and the birth control methods they are using. By means of monthly visits to the home of each woman of "childbearing age," which is defined as the time of marriage to menopause, the Red Medical Workers keep careful track of the contraceptives used. A chart on the wall at the Silvery Lane health station outlines the birth control methods used in the lane (Table 7). Abortions are free and easily available but are almost never requested by unmarried women; we were told that pregnancies among unmarried women are exceedingly rare; out-of-wedlock births are essentially unheard of. The annual crude birth rate in Silvery Lane was reported to be at the almost incredibly low level of 5.9 per 1,000 population.

In Kung Chiang New Village, part of the Yang Pu District in the industrial northeast section of Shanghai, we talked with the Red Medical Workers conducting family planning education at the residents' committee level. All of these trained housewives, each with two or three children, had had tubal ligations, so

TABLE 7. FAMILY PLANNING CHART IN THE SILVERY LANE HEALTH
STATION, HANGCHOW, SERVING 2,700 PEOPLE, SEPTEMBER 1971

	Number	Percent of Total
Total number of married woman of childbearing age	369	100
Vasectomies	10	3
Tubal ligation	89	24
Total permanently sterilized	99	27
Oral contraceptives	65	17
Condom	69	19
IUD	22	6
Rhythm	7	2
Other	9	2
Total using contraceptives	172	46
Husband outside the city	21	6
"Has not been pregnant"	6	2
Breast feeding	16	4
Newly married	7	2
Chronically ill	13	3
Other	25	7
Total not using contraceptives	88	24
Pregnant	10	3

Abortions, January-September 1971: None
Birth Rate, January-September 1971: 5.9 per 1,000

they served as models for the women they visited monthly. They
told us that while no one was "forced" to limit the family to two
or three children, they put great stress on educating people on
the importance—not necessarily to themselves, but rather to
Shanghai and to China—of population control. As a result of
these intensive neighborhood campaigns the crude birth rate
for the city proper of Shanghai in 1971 was approximately 7 per
1,000, and 6.1 per 1,000 in the first three months of 1972. Supporting evidence for this extremely low rate—lower than the
crude death rate of 6.4 per 1,000 in the first three months of

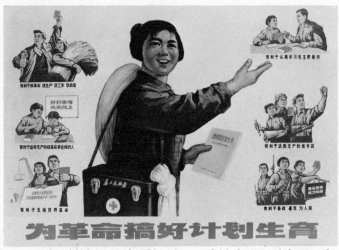

Poster urging birth control: "Plan for good birth control for revolution." A barefoot doctor holds a book entitled, *Late Marriage and Plan for Birth Control: Collection of Information and Experience.* Her medical bag is inscribed, *Wei renmin fuwu,* "Serve the People." The captions around the periphery give reasons for practicing "planned birth." Starting at the upper right hand corner, they are: 1) In order to study and apply Chairman Mao's Thought in a lively way; 2) in order to consolidate the proletarian dictatorship; 3) in order to prepare against war, prepare against national disaster, and for the people; 4) in order to support world revolution; (the poster in the hands of the workers reads, "People of the whole world unite to defeat the American imperialists and all their running dogs"—Mao Tsetung); 5) in order to cultivate successors to the proletarian revolution; (the sign behind the teacher and student reads, "Study well and make progress every day"); and 6) in order to grasp revolution, promote production, carry on work, and prepare against war.

1972, with a consequent negative rate of natural population growth—is provided by the 1971 census of the Luwan district of Shanghai and other data described in Appendix E.

Sian, the capital of Shensi Province in the midwest, with a population of 2.4 million, is divided into five districts, one of which is Lian Hu in the central west section. Within the Lian Hu district is the "city commune" or neighborhood of Ching Nian, organized in 1958 during the Great Leap Forward, with a population of 40,000; it, in turn, is divided into twenty-six residents' committees. In the east section of Ching Nian Lu (Youth Road) live 302 families totaling 1,022 people whose routine medical needs are met by five Red Medical Workers operating out of a health station situated in the midst of the neighborhood.

The health station consists of two rooms, each about fifteen feet square, on either side of a courtyard. One room is used primarily for treatment and for the storage of medications and acupuncture equipment. Posters brighten the white concrete walls; one, a quotation from Chairman Mao, reads: "We must call on the masses to arise in struggle against their own illiteracy, superstitions and unhygienic habits." The second room is used for examining patients and for conferences.

Of the seventeen patients we observed being examined and treated by the Red Medical Workers, all wearing white coats and working together in the examination room, sixteen were women and one was a retired male worker. The patients complained of a variety of symptoms:

—A female factory worker had had abdominal pains off and on for five or six years, and came to the health station regularly for acupuncture treatment; she used to take yeast tablets, but felt that acupuncture was better. She was treated with four acupuncture needles in the abdomen and one in the right foot.

—A female patient with chronic hepatitis had medicine prescribed at the commune hospital and brought it to the health station every other day for injection. Each injection cost her five *fen*.

—A sixty-four-year-old man with high blood pressure wanted his pressure measured. It was 190/100 and no change in his medication was made. Since he was a retired worker, there was no charge for the visit.

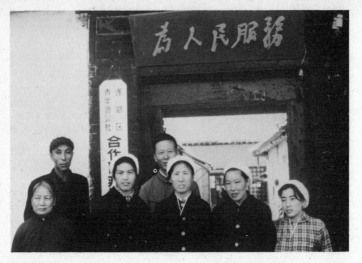

Red Medical Workers and members of the revolutionary committee, Ching Nian Lu residents' committee, Sian. Sign over entrance to the health station reads: *Wei renmin fuwu,* "Serve the People."

Patients are referred from the Ching Nian Lu health station to the Ching Nian commune hospital, which has eight departments—medicine, surgery, acupuncture, traditional medicine, ophthalmology, massage, gynecology and obstetrics, and X-ray—and a laboratory. The hospital is open Monday through Saturday, on Wednesday and Friday evenings, and on Sundays for emergencies only. The hospital's ten doctors—three traditional and seven Western-trained—and twenty-one nurses see 400 to 500 patients daily.

Dr. Sing Yu-ying, of the Department of Internal Medicine, treats patients with hypertension, upper respiratory infections, bronchitis, dysentery, gastritis and enteritis, hepatitis, and kidney and neurological diseases. He also sees some cases of ascariasis and pinworm. Patients with heart disease or cancer, said to be relatively rare, are referred to the Second Municipal Hospital, as are patients with dehydration due to gastrointestinal disorders.

Urban Hospitals

Hospitals in the cities range from technologically sophisticated research and teaching hospitals to small neighborhood "hospitals" that care only for ambulatory patients. In Peking, there are four research-oriented and specialized hospitals operated under the aegis of the Academy of Medical Sciences (AMS); twenty-three municipal hospitals, ten of which have over 500 beds, under the jurisdiction of the Peking Bureau of Public Health; and twenty district hospitals. The hospitals run by the AMS are the Shoutu, the Fu Wai, the Jih Tan (a tumor hospital), and a dermatology institute.

The Shoutu (Capital) Hospital, formerly the hospital of the Peking Union Medical College, was called the Fanti (Anti-Imperialist) Hospital from the onset of the Cultural Revolution until early 1972 when it was renamed. It is a general facility of 550 beds, which also cares for about 2,000 patients a day in its clinics. The hospital has a staff of 900 including 215 doctors, 335 nurses, and sixty-nine pharmacists, technicians, and other intermediate-level medical personnel. A list of the current department chairmen and other staff, and information on the whereabouts of former staff members, is given in Appendix F. The buildings of Peking Union Medical College, widely acclaimed at the time of their construction as an architectural feat combining traditional Chinese and Western styles, now have a banner over the main entrance reading *Wei renmin fuwu*—"Serve the People."

During our visit in 1972 the vice-chairman of the revolutionary committee of the hospital, the chairman of the Department of Medicine, and other members of the staff described the four tasks of the hospital:

1. *Treatment:* The hospital serves as the referral hospital for thirty-seven units—factories, shops, and offices. Patients with serious problems are referred to the hospital from every province of China, and the doctors travel, often in mobile medical teams, to distant provinces to provide care. In the fall of 1972 there were four mobile teams in the countryside and border areas.

2. *Education:* The hospital currently provides postgraduate speciality training for eighty physicians. It is also training 120

nursing students in a course which, since the Cultural Revolution, takes two years. In addition, doctors trained in Western medicine spend eight months full-time in the hospital learning traditional medicine.

3. *Research:* The hospital conducts a full program of research under the auspices of the AMS. Research fields include chronic bronchitis, coronary heart disease, cancer (including carcinoma of the breast, chorioepithelioma, and leukemia), contraception, and acupuncture anesthesia. The superb library of the academy is located in one wing of the hospital.

4. *Treatment of Foreign Visitors:* The hospital treats visitors and diplomatic personnel from the Western capitalist countries. It was the site of James Reston's well-publicized appendectomy in 1971.

The Fu Chen Men Wai Hospital, also known as Fu Wai Hospital, specializes in chest and heart diseases; 60 to 70 per cent of its 350 beds are devoted to cardiology. The Jih Tan Hospital is associated with the Tumor Institute of the AMS. The dermatology institute was said to have been moved to the countryside during the Cultural Revolution.

The twenty-three municipal hospitals sponsored by the Bureau of Public Health include the Gong-Nong-Bing (Worker-Peasant-Soldier), the Chishueit'an, the Third Teaching Hospital attached to the Peking Medical College, and the Youyi (Friendship) Hospital. The Gong-Nong-Bing Hospital has 600 beds and a staff of 1,000, including 300 doctors and 250 nurses; specialties include ophthalmology and otolaryngology. The Chishueit'an Hospital has 500 beds and a staff that includes 215 doctors and about 300 nurses; among its specialties are orthopedics and the treatment of burns and other traumas. It handles 3,000 outpatient visits and 350 emergency room visits daily. The Third Teaching Hospital, which we visited in 1971, has 600 beds and a staff of 600.

The Youyi Hospital, which we also visited in 1971 and learned more about in 1972 from Dr. Chang Wei-hsun (Arthur Chang), its deputy director, specializes in internal medicine. Of its total of 805 beds, 195 are assigned to medicine. It has thirteen

clinical departments: anesthesiology, dermatology, general surgery, medicine, neurology, neurosurgery, obstetrics-gynecology,
ophthalmology, orthopedics, otolaryngology, pediatrics, stomatology, and urology. In addition there are a number of "auxiliary"
departments, such as the Department of Radioisotopes and Radiology, and research laboratories. Of the staff of 1,032, 260 are
doctors, 254 are nurses, and sixty-seven are technicians.

In the immediate community of 90,000 people served by
Youyi Hospital, there are ninety-three local "units," including
factories and schools. The hospital also has responsibility for four
lane health stations and seven district hospitals, and acts as the
referral center for a rural county of Peking. The total population
cared for is therefore much larger—approximately 700,000.

The hospital was built in 1952 with Soviet help, and was
originally named the Sino-Soviet Friendship Hospital. From the
beginning of the Cultural Revolution until 1971 it was called the
Anti-Revisionist Hospital. Youyi Hospital renders medical care
to visitors to China from the socialist countries.

In Shanghai we visited the city's largest hospital, which has
1,100 beds. During our 1971 visit it was called the Dongfanghong
(East Is Red) Hospital; by the time of our 1972 visit it had been
renamed the Juichin Hospital, for the street on which it is located.
Built in 1907, it was originally a French Jesuit hospital affiliated
with Aurora Medical School. At the time the government took it
over in 1952, we were told, it had 700 beds, and the staff consisted
of thirty doctors, forty nurses, and 230 other workers. It now
has a total staff of 1,400, including 300 doctors, 400 nurses, and
160 technicians.

The hospital's active ambulatory service cares for 3,000 patients daily; the emergency room serves approximately 300 adults
and 100 children a day. The inpatient service has a 92 per cent
occupancy rate and admits about 15,000 patients a year. It is
therefore possible to calculate a mean length of stay of approximately twenty-five days, at a cost per day of about 1 *yüan* (U.S.
40 cents). The hospital's annual budget, exclusive of food, is
approximately 3 million *yüan* ($1 million).

Juichin Hospital is one of the four teaching units of the Shanghai Second Medical College, the others being Gong-Nong-Bing, Xinhua (New China), and the Shanghai Ninth Municipal hospitals. Medical students, interns, residents, and postgraduate students are trained at Juichin.

At the other end of Shanghai's hospital spectrum is the Kung Chiang neighborhood hospital in the Yangpu district, which we visited in 1972. Each of the eleven residents' committees of the neighborhood has a cooperative health station staffed by Red Medical Workers under the supervision of doctors from the neighborhood hospital. Patients are referred from the health stations to the hospital, which has no inpatient beds but serves an average of 800 ambulatory patients daily. The hospital employs eighty-eight people, of whom sixty-four are "medical personnel." Among these there are twelve graduates of regular medical college, nine assistant doctors, five traditional doctors, approximately thirty nurses, a pharmacist, a dentist, and an X-ray technician.

In the pediatrics department we observed a regular medical college graduate and an assistant doctor examining patients in the same room and apparently consulting together regularly. The Department of Traditional Medicine sees over 100 patients a day who choose to consult its doctors. The hospital is administered by a six-member revolutionary committee, composed of three medical personnel, all of whom at the time of our visit happened to be nurses, and three administrators, one of whom is a member of the propaganda team from one of the factories of the district.

HEALTH CARE IN URBAN FACTORIES

China's factories have highly organized medical services and are major sites of health care in the urban areas. Most factories have a central clinic as well as health stations in individual workshops; often there is a factory hospital with beds for short-term stays. The worker doctor is the analogue in the factories of the Red Medical Worker and the barefoot doctor; just as a peasant is chosen by his peers to become a barefoot doctor, a factory employee is chosen by his fellow workers to become a worker doctor. The formal training seems in general to be shorter than that of the barefoot doctor and a little longer than that of

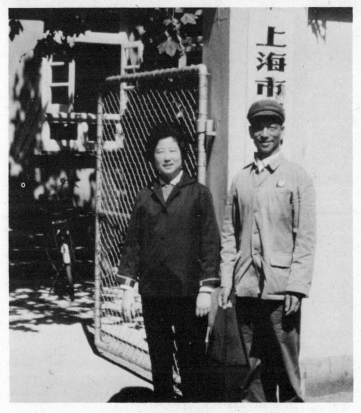

Nurse and neighborhood worker, members of the revolutionary committee, Kung Chiang neighborhood hospital, Shanghai.

the Red Medical Worker, usually taking about a month. Continuing on-the-job supervision and training is considered extremely important.

The worker doctor has the responsibility for health education, preventive medicine, and the treatment of minor complaints, which he often takes care of right in the workshop. He usually spends a specific period of time in the factory hospital or clinic where he receives continuing supervision and training by fully-trained, full-time doctors.

Liu Chung-sun, twenty-eight years old and a worker doctor in a Peking handicraft factory, is a fairly typical example. Two years ago, after working for ten years in the factory, he received one month's training as a worker doctor. Since then his continuing training consists of spending one day every two weeks in his factory's clinic. When his production schedule permits, he spends a week in the clinic giving such treatments as subcutaneous, intramuscular, and intravenous injections under supervision.

In his workshop Comrade Liu has responsibility for about forty workers, but is called on to give medical care only once or twice a week. The bulk of his health work is spent on health education and preventive medicine. He teaches his fellow workers to recognize the early signs of certain diseases such as hypertension and hepatitis; as a preventive measure against the latter he urges the washing of hands before meals and after using the toilet. Other preventive measures include making certain that the immunizations of the workers in his shop are up-to-date, and attempting to limit the spread of infections.

"Common illnesses" are treated by Comrade Liu in the shop, most often by the use of acupuncture. Among the disorders he treats are the common cold, headache, backache, ankle sprain, and gastroenteritis. He told us that for headache he gets results from acupuncture in about two minutes in about 80 per cent of his patients, and that he thinks it is more effective than aspirin or APC (aspirin-phenacetin-caffeine).

Comrade Liu told us frankly that there are certain symptoms about which the workers do not consult him; they either confer among themselves or take the problem directly to the clinic. In the case of dysmenorrhea, for example, the women usually exchange information and one of them may then ask him for a particular remedy another woman has recommended. The medications we found in Comrade Liu's medicine cabinet are listed in Appendix G. As we reviewed them, he seemed to have a firm knowledge of the nature of the medications, their indications and contraindications, and the kinds of adverse reactions that should be watched for.

The Third Textile Mill of Peking, which we visited in 1971, employs over 6,000 workers. Seventy full-time medical personnel staff the clinic and a thirty-bed hospital for the workers and their families. The clinic provides medical, surgical, and obstetrical services. Uncomplicated deliveries are performed in the hospital; complicated deliveries are referred to the municipal hospital. Preventive measures include periodic checkups of workers and regular exercise periods during the workday.

At the Fengsheng Neighborhood Insulation Material Factory in Peking, Tung Shih-ping, a shy, soft-spoken young woman of eighteen is the worker doctor to 190 workers. Comrade Tung attended primary school for six years and middle school for three years, graduating in 1970. She came to work in the factory in July of the same year, and shortly thereafter was chosen by the

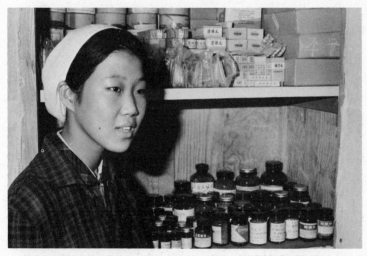

Tung Shih-ping, worker doctor, Fengsheng Neighborhood Insulation Material Factory, Peking. On the top shelf are traditional Chinese medicines, on the bottom, Western-type medicines.

factory's revolutionary committee to be trained as a medical worker. Starting in November 1970 she was trained at the People's Hospital for three months.

Comrade Tung told us she does "mainly preventive work, some sanitation work, and treats 'light disease.' " She takes blood pressures and temperatures, and has a variety of medicines, similar to those of the worker doctor in the Peking handicraft factory, with which to treat minor illnesses. The medicine cabinet in the small room that serves as her medical station is filled with approximately fifty Western medicines and forty traditional medicines. If there is an emergency Comrade Tung will refer the worker to the Fengsheng neighborhood hospital; if the patient fails to improve he will be referred to the district-level People's Hospital. Patients with certain illnesses can be referred directly to a specialty hospital.

Comrade Tung also does family planning work among the women workers in the factory. She stressed that birth control is a matter of free choice, but that she tries to educate the women about family planning. If a woman has one girl and one boy, Comrade Tung told us she encourages the woman to use the pill, which she provides, or have an intrauterine device inserted in People's Hospital. "However, if the woman has two girls, she usually wants to have another child to try for a boy."

The Peking Printing and Dyeing Mill is a much larger factory that produces an average of 80 million meters of printed cotton a year. Forty-four medical workers—two Western-trained doctors, four assistant doctors, one pharmacist, nine nurses, and twenty-eight worker doctors—are available to care for 2,000 workers and their families. The two doctors attended regular medical colleges, and the four assistant doctors attended middle medical colleges. The salary for fully-trained doctors ranges from 46 *yüan* a month for a beginning doctor to 170 *yüan* a month for the most experienced. The assistant doctors' salaries begin at 32 *yüan* a month, as do the nurses' salaries, and rise to 80 *yüan* a month.

The worker doctors, on the other hand, are paid at the same rate as regular workers on a scale ranging from 34 *yüan* a month for the beginner to 240 *yüan* for the most experienced. The

twenty-eight worker doctors were trained for three months, full-
time, in a People's Liberation Army hospital in 1969 and have
since had training in ear, nose, throat, and eye diseases, and in
traditional Chinese medicine in specialty hospitals. They were
chosen by their fellow workers and received full pay during their
training period.

All workers at the factory have an annual physical examination, which includes a chest X-ray. Female workers, in addition,
have annual vaginal smears and breast examinations. Special
attention is paid to the blood pressure of workers in high tem-
perature shops. Cooks in the factory dining hall and nursery
school teachers have screening tests for hepatitis and stool
examinations for ova and parasites, in addition to the regular
examination. The children in the nursery are not given routine
physical examinations at the factory, but do receive their immunizations there.

Since the factory operates on a three-shift, twenty-four-hour-
day basis, medical personnel are on round-the-clock duty. The
factory is closed on Sunday, but a medical worker is on duty in
case the maintenance men need care.

The medical facilities are separate from the factory, in con-
necting one-story, one-room units that consist of departments
of internal medicine, ENT, obstetrics and gynecology, surgery,
and acupuncture, a laboratory, a treatment room, a pharmacy
with traditional and Western medicines, and a simple ward in
which patients may stay overnight or possibly as long as a week
for diagnostic purposes.

In the "women's" department, of the twenty examinations
done on an average day, fifteen are prenatal tests. Up to the
seventh month, a pregnant woman is examined once a month;
from the seventh month on, every two weeks; and during the last
month, at weekly intervals. The examinations routinely include
the taking of blood pressure, screening for anemia, urinalysis, and
assessment of the fetal position. At the end of her fifty-six-day
maternity leave, the mother is examined before returning to
work. Deliveries usually take place in the Peking Women's
Hospital.

If workers are away from the factory due to illness for only a day or two, they are not examined when they come back. If a worker is ill for a longer period of time, however, he is examined upon his return. The medical workers estimated that 5.5 per cent of the workers are absent for at least one day a month due to illness; on a typical day the absentee rate is roughly 1 per cent, an extremely low rate compared with that for Western countries.

PAYMENT FOR MEDICAL CARE

Methods of payment for care in the cities vary widely, from total subsidization by the patient's factory to payment by the patient for individual services. An official 1963 Peking publication, *For the Health of the People,* stated:

> Free medical care is extended to government employees, industrial workers, miners, university and college students, and to the entire population in some of the national minority areas. To those who are unable to pay for treatment, the local authorities . . . grant allowances according to their specific conditions.[3]

During our visits we were told that workers in most industries have all medical care paid for by their factories; their families are subsidized for half the cost of the services and must pay the balance themselves. The workers at the printing and dyeing factory pay neither a registration fee nor a fee for medical care for work-related illness; for non-work-related illness they pay only the 5 *fen* registration fee. Members of a worker's family must pay the registration fee plus half the cost of the medicine. We were told, however, that families generally do not use the factory facilities; they are apt to use medical facilities more convenient to their residences or in their own place of employment.

In Kwangchow, urban "cooperative medical care systems" are being tried experimentally. By contributing 1 *yüan* a month, the patient's ambulatory care is given free at the time of service, and only one-tenth of the cost of inpatient care is paid directly by the patient.

The Chinese hope to see the elimination of all medical care payments "when there are sufficient resources to make this possible." Apparently this will be done, as is so much else, on a decentralized basis. The cost of individual service and of pre-payment premiums is extremely low, not only by American standards but as a percentage of a Chinese worker's income; the payments are therefore felt to be little or no barrier to access to care.

NOTES

1. Leo A. Orleans, *Every Fifth Child: The Population of China* (Stanford: Stanford University Press, 1972): p. 49.

2. Han Suyin, "Family Planning in China," in *Population and Family Planning in the People's Republic of China,* ed., Phyllis T. Piotrow (New York: Victor-Bostrom Fund and Population Crisis Committee, 1971): pp. 16-21.

3. *For the Health of the People* (Peking: Foreign Languages Press, 1963): pp. 2-3.

III. Health Care in
the Countryside

RURAL CHINA

IN order to understand the current organization of health services in the Chinese countryside it is necessary to have some knowledge of certain aspects of rural life. China is still a predominantly rural nation—we were told that 80 per cent of the people live in the "countryside." While the definitions on which such urban-rural statistics are based are not totally clear, the significance of the data can be appreciated when they are contrasted with those of other countries of comparable size. In the United States, for example, only 27 per cent of the population live in what the Bureau of the Census in 1970 defined as rural areas; [1] in the Soviet Union the figure is 44 per cent; [2] in India it is 82 per cent. [3]

In some ways even more important than the total number of people living outside the cities is their distribution. As noted in the introduction to this volume, most of the population is concentrated in eastern China. The provision of adequate services to the rural population is therefore complicated not only by their vast numbers but by areas of relatively high and of exceedingly low population densities.

Before Liberation the paucity of resources available to the rural population was further exacerbated by the despotic landlord and warlord systems that deprived the peasants of remuneration for their toil on the land and even of an adequate share of the food they produced. One of the first priorities in each liberated area therefore was for the peasants themselves to distribute the land among those who worked and lived on it.* In the period following Liberation the land and the primitive tools for working it thus became the property of individual peasants.

During the 1950s groups with increasingly collective ownership called "cooperatives" were formed. By the late 1950s and early 1960s much of the farmland had been converted into communes, with collective ownership of agricultural tools and of the land, except for small private plots on which the peasants could grow food for personal consumption. The communes were often large enough to include all the households of a township, whose government was then combined with the management of the commune. Unlike the cooperatives, which were purely economic organizations, the communes became units of both political and economic organization. Their members' "representative assemblies" function as the townships' "people's congresses." Today communes are formal, self-contained political units with their own internal governments, usually reporting directly to the government of the county in which they are located.

The smallest subdivision of the commune is the "production team," with a membership of several hundred people. The team leadership is responsible for the day-to-day planning of the team's work. People on the same production team live close to one another, usually in small villages, and form the basic social unit in the countryside. Several teams combine to form a "production brigade," which usually has wider responsibility than the team with regard to health, transportation, and, in the north, the grinding and storing of grain. A typical commune is composed of ten to thirty production brigades. The commune is the lowest level of formal state power in the rural areas, analogous to the "neighborhoods" in the cities, and is responsible for overall planning, education, health and social services, and the operation of small factories that produce goods for its members and for outside distribution.

Despite the vast changes that took place in the countryside

* This process, an understanding of which is in our view crucial to an understanding of China today, has been vividly described by William Hinton in his book, *Fanshen*.[4]

from 1949 to 1965, the Chinese with whom we spoke felt that the rural areas had not advanced at the same rate as the urban areas. Following the Soviet pattern, great stress was placed on urban industrialization during that period. Material incentives were given, particularly in the cities, to those who produced more or did better work. A large wage differential grew up between the highest-paid managers and technicians, on the one hand, and the factory workers, on the other. A managerial elite emerged, and selected people in the society had greater wealth and more material possessions than did others.

As the Chinese now describe it, an increasingly large group of people had no memories of the "bitter past" or of the Long March, and had lost much of the spirit of the struggle which led to Liberation in 1949. As a result, we were told, the managerial elite largely lost touch with the people they were supposed to serve, favored industrialization of the cities over the strengthening of the rural areas, and forgot the meaning of hard physical work and self-reliance.

In health services this took the form of improvement of the "quality" of the services by the development of urban medical centers. While some health personnel were indeed assigned to the countryside, the major effort appeared to lie in strengthening medical care in the cities in the hope that some would spill over into the rural areas. But doctors and other health workers, most of them recruited from the cities where adequate secondary education was available, were largely unwilling—as in other countries—to move into the poorer and culturally more barren countryside.

THE DEVELOPMENT OF THE BAREFOOT DOCTOR

With medical care in the countryside lagging behind that in the cities, and with a clearly inadequate supply of doctors to meet the needs of all the people, efforts began in the late 1950s to train indigenous rural personnel who would participate in agricultural production and at the same time deliver health care.* For

---

* There were precedents for this type of training in China; John Grant, for example, described the training of comparable rural "medical helpers" in the 1920s and 1930s.[5]

example, in 1958, as part of the Great Leap Forward, physicians
in Shanghai organized themselves to go to nearby rural areas

> . . . where, in cooperation with the clinics of the people's com-
> munes, they trained in short-term classes and through practice,
> large numbers of health workers who did not divorce themselves
> from production. Figures for June 1960 show that there were over
> 3,900 such health workers in the more than 2,500 production bri-
> gades of the ten counties under the Shanghai municipality.[6]

During the period 1961–65 there was said to have been a
cessation of training and a reduction in the number of such
health workers. A report, now criticized as "revisionist," "counterrevolutionary," and "malicious," was issued that condemned the
role of the health workers in the production brigades and suggested
that it would be better if they dropped their medical work and
devoted themselves to agricultural tasks. The 3,900 health workers
in the Shanghai counties were therefore reduced in number to
just over 300. In the months immediately preceding the Cultural
Revolution the training of rural health workers was apparently
resumed, and by the time Mao Tse-tung issued his "June 26th
Directive" in 1965 the number of health workers in production
brigades of the Shanghai counties had increased to more than
2,300.

The training of barefoot doctors began in earnest following
Mao's directive. Still using the Shanghai countryside as the example, by 1968 there were 4,500 barefoot doctors who themselves had
trained more than 29,000 peasants as auxiliary "health workers"
for the production teams. In 1971 we were told that the 2,724
production brigades in the rural counties of the Shanghai
municipality were served by 7,702 barefoot doctors. Their number
had apparently increased markedly throughout China, for there
are now said to be "over a million" barefoot doctors and the
Chinese are very proud of their work. Unlike the attitude of
Soviet health officials, for example, who are attempting to "phase
out" workers such as the feldsher,[7] or at least give them a more
limited, technical, subordinate role,[8] the Chinese with whom we
talked felt that the barefoot doctor is playing an indispensable
role in health care and is likely to continue to do so for many
years to come.

The term "barefoot doctor" (*chijiao yisheng*) loses much in translation—as it turned out, every barefoot doctor with whom we spoke was wearing shoes. The word *chijiao*, barefoot, is used to emphasize that he is indeed a peasant, which is not a derogatory term in China, rather than to describe his lack of footwear. To quote directly from a definition provided in English by the Chinese themselves: "A 'barefoot doctor' is a peasant who has had basic medical training and gives treatment without leaving productive work. He gets the name because in the south peasants work barefooted in rice paddies." [9] The reader should also not be confused by the translation of *yisheng* as "doctor," which it indeed means in other contexts. Chinese officials do not equate the *chijiao yisheng* with regularly trained doctors: the former are counted in statistics as peasants rather than as health workers. Their patients similarly are said to understand the differences. They refer to their barefoot doctor not as *yisheng* or *daifu* (which also means doctor), but as *tongzhi* (comrade), the common form of address for everyone in China including doctors. In short, the four Chinese characters in combination that translate as "barefoot doctor" take on a set of denotations and connotations that are lost in literal translation. It might be preferable in English to use the term "peasant doctor" [10] or "peasant health worker," but we will use "barefoot doctor" because that is the common PRC English designation.

STATUS AND PAYMENT OF THE BAREFOOT DOCTOR

Since the barefoot doctor is a peasant, in planting and harvesting seasons almost all of his time is spent in farming work. In slack periods, however, a considerable part, often more than half, of his time is spent catching up on the health needs of his production brigade, particularly in the areas of environmental control and preventive medicine.

The barefoot doctor is considered by his community, and apparently thinks of himself, as a peasant who performs some medical duties rather than as a health worker who does some agricultural work. Herein, as well as in length and content of training and in certain aspects of the job description, lies the difference between the barefoot doctor and the Soviet rural feldsher.[11, 12] The feldsher is clearly thought of, and thinks of himself, as a health worker in rural practice. As a result he feels put upon if he is required to do any nonmedical work. The view was effectively presented in a 1968 story, "Hay Is Our Main Concern," in *Krokodil*, the Soviet satirical journal.[13] In this story, the feldshers are required to cut grain to feed their own horses, a task they obviously consider a waste of their time and medical training, as well as—though it is not explicitly stated—below their dignity.

Neither should the barefoot doctors be confused with the medical assistants of certain countries of Africa and the South Pacific who, like feldshers, spend essentially full time in health and medical care [14] and are separated in a number of tangible and intangible ways from the people they serve. Few parallels to the barefoot doctors exist in other countries; where they do exist they are usually called "auxiliaries." [15]

Despite the fact that he spends much of his time doing medical work, the barefoot doctor receives the usual wages of an agricultural worker. A commune member's income depends on the total income of his commune and the number of work points he collects. The barefoot doctor generates his work points by doing medical work just as though he had been doing agricultural work during the same period. Like his fellow commune workers, he receives an equal share of the distributed produce of the commune, and cash from its sale of produce based on the number of work points he has collected.

As a peasant, the barefoot doctor's income is lower than that of the doctors working on the commune, who are not considered to be peasants. Beginning doctors now earn a salary on the order of 600 *yüan* (about U.S. $240) a year compared to the 300 *yüan* or less earned annually in cash by the peasants, including the barefoot doctors. Since the cash income of the barefoot doctor and other commune members is supplemented by distribution of produce, however, and since the cost of living in the communes is said to be much lower than in the urban areas, the differences may be less marked than they appear.

The Training of the Barefoot Doctor

As in the current recruitment of medical students in China, barefoot doctor trainees are chosen by those whom they will serve. Political ideology and a desire to "serve the people" are said to be of major importance in their selection; while these are ideologic qualities, we received the impression that the teams and brigades are attempting to select individuals who genuinely wanted to care for others. All the barefoot doctors with whom we spoke mentioned the honor they felt on being chosen for training by their fellow production team or brigade members.

Just as much of the work of the barefoot doctor seems to vary from place to place, so too does the pattern of his education. Formal training ranges from three- or four-month periods in successive years, interspersed with on-the-job supervision and guidance, to a single three- to six-month period of training followed by a variable period of on-the-job supervised experience. The formal training period is usually taken in a county or commune hospital and is fairly evenly divided between theoretical and practical work. As seems to be true of most job requirements in present-day China, there appears to be little emphasis on particular duration or type of training, and even less on earning a specific credential or degree; rather, it is on the skills an individual demonstrates in a particular job situation.

As a concrete example of a training pattern, consider the Sing Sing Production Brigade of the Horse Bridge Commune outside of Shanghai consisting of 1,850 people, which in 1971 was served by four barefoot doctors and one midwife. Ho Shi-chang, the eldest of the barefoot doctors, is thirty years of age. His formal education prior to becoming a barefoot doctor consisted of six years of primary school, which he completed at age thirteen. In 1964, when he was twenty-one, he received three months of formal medical training from doctors in the county hospital—there were thirteen doctors to teach a class of 274 students—and a further three months of practical training in the commune hospital, where he now spends one day a week for continuing education.

The second barefoot doctor, Chang Dao-jing, is twenty-six

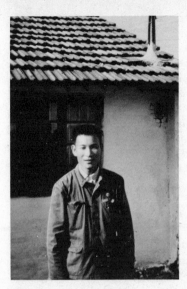

Left: Ho Shi-chang, barefoot doctor, Sing Sing Production Brigade, Shanghai.

Below: Health station, Sing Sing Production Brigade. Kao Ning-shin, brigade midwife, is seen on the right.

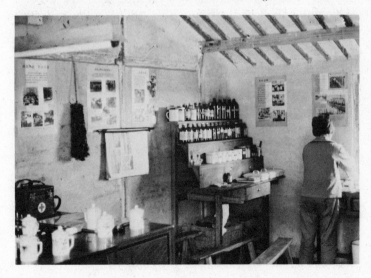

and received his training at the commune hospital in 1965 at the age of eighteen. Chow Sing, the third barefoot doctor, is now twenty-four and was formally trained at the commune hospital for three months in 1968 at the age of nineteen. The sixty students in his class were trained by both regular doctors and barefoot doctors. Half of the training was devoted to theory and half to practical experience. Like Ho, Chow goes once a week to the commune hospital and health station where he spends half the day in class and the other half taking care of patients under supervision. Hao Wen-shio, the fourth barefoot doctor, is twenty-three years of age; she too was trained at the commune hospital in 1968 at the age of eighteen.

Kao Ning-shin, the brigade midwife, is thirty-three. In 1966 at age twenty-six she received a three-month midwifery course at the county hospital. She usually performs two or three deliveries a month and returns to the county hospital one day a month for further training.

The training and responsibilities of Liu Yu-sheng, the twenty-eight-year-old barefoot doctor of the Double North Production Team (population 509) of the Double Bridge People's Commune near Peking are also fairly typical. After graduating from junior middle school Liu worked in the production team as a peasant. When in 1965 Chairman Mao issued his June 26th directive to put stress on medical care in the rural areas, Liu was elected by the members of the team to be trained as a barefoot doctor. He was trained for three months in his commune by mobile teams of doctors from urban hospitals. Since he began his work Comrade Liu has had short leaves of absence for further study, and recently he went to Peking for three months to study traditional Chinese medicine. He focuses on prevention, health education, and the treatment of "common diseases."

As with the educational pattern of regular doctors, there is said to be little stress on grades and competition among the students. Each is expected to help fellow students who may be slower at learning the material or the techniques. In any event, since each barefoot doctor returns to his own production brigade to work, there would appear to be little advantage in scoring academic points. The impetus for learning comes from the students' recognition that they will be responsible for the health of their fellow workers after they return to the commune; this, we were told, provides the incentive to learn, rather than examinations or grades.

On returning to the commune there apparently follows a period of fairly closely supervised work. An example of this was given us by Dr. Hsu Chia-yu, deputy chief of internal medicine at the Juichin Hospital in Shanghai, who was our interpreter during our first trip. He told us of training barefoot doctors in a county hospital and then returning with them to their communes to provide on-the-job supervision and training. Dr. Hsu described how he lived with a barefoot doctor and his family, sleeping in the same bed with him and using the same pillow. He said this had been quite difficult for him because he had been raised in Shanghai and had never shared a pillow with anyone before. Dr. Hsu described how he and the barefoot doctor, before going to sleep, would talk about the patients they had seen during the day and their hopes and goals for their society.

A most important part of the training is felt to be the barefoot doctor's regular work with trained doctors in the commune hospital and health center. The nature of this training varies from commune to commune, ranging from the barefoot doctor spending one day a week to as little as one day a month at the center.

THE BAREFOOT DOCTOR'S DUTIES

As with his training, the barefoot doctor's duties vary from area to area, commune to commune, and even brigade to brigade within the same commune. There are, however, many standard activities. In general they have responsibility for environmental sanitation, health education, immunizations, first aid, and aspects of personal primary medical care and post-illness follow-up.

With regard to environmental sanitation the barefoot doctor is responsible, for example, for the proper collection, treatment, storage, and use of human feces as fertilizer. While these tasks are usually carried out by health workers whom he has trained, the work is inspected regularly by the barefoot doctor. He is also responsible for directing campaigns against such pests as flies, cockroaches, fleas, or snails, and he or the health workers visit the homes of commune members regularly to spray insecticides. His health education efforts include teaching hygiene to his fellow commune members.

Immunizations are an important responsibility of the barefoot doctor, although again they are often done by the health workers under supervision. At the health center of the Mai Chia Wu Production Brigade of the West Lake People's Commune near Hangchow, Mai Jen-chai, one of the brigade's two barefoot doctors, showed us the detailed immunization records for each child in the 251 families of the brigade: as in the cities, the immunizations were for diphtheria, pertussis, poliomyelitis, measles, smallpox, meningococcal meningitis, and Japanese B encephalitis.

The barefoot doctor is usually readily available for medical emergencies since he normally works in the fields with his patients and lives among them. Comrade Mai told us that he treats colds, bronchitis, gastrointestinal disorders, measles, and minor injuries; more complicated problems are referred to the commune health station. The auxiliary health worker also plays a role; he can apply dressings for minor injuries and give medication for headaches, colds, and fever.

Hsiao Hsiu-yun, a twenty-two-year-old shy yet enthusiastic barefoot doctor at the Taipingchiao Production Brigade of the China-Rumania Friendship People's Commune southwest of Peking, was trained in the commune hospital for three months beginning in January 1970. She and thirteen other barefoot doctors care for the "light diseases" of the brigade's 2,900 people.* They take turns staffing the sparsely furnished, three-room brigade health station from 7:30 A.M. to noon, and again from 2:30 to 7:00 P.M. In addition, one of them is always on duty at the health

* This commune, with a population of 46,000, had trained 450 barefoot doctors. That ratio of approximately 1:100 (or 1:200 in the Taipingchiao brigade) was the highest we observed in China. The 7,702 barefoot doctors in the rural areas of the Shanghai municipality, for example, serve 4.7 million people, a ratio of about 1:600; the latter ratio is more consistent with the overall estimate of "1 million" barefoot doctors for China's 750-800 million people.

station during the lunch break, after seven in the evening, and all night.

These barefoot doctors immunize all the brigade's children from the ages of one to seven; the immunization records are kept on cards in the health station and are filed according to production team. While the brigade midwife delivers the babies, Comrade Hsiao told us that the barefoot doctors are responsible for educating the brigade women about family planning and providing them with contraceptives. The barefoot doctors plant traditional Chinese medicinal herbs, go to the mountains to collect additional herbs, make up pills, and prepare injections and fill and label the vials.

In the communes we visited, the brigade midwife, invariably a woman, had received training similar to that of the barefoot doctor and has equal status. She provides prenatal care and health education, and performs uncomplicated deliveries. Midwives give special attention to education in, and encouragement in the use of, birth control methods.

Some idea of the range of knowledge the barefoot doctor is supposed to acquire is given in the several different versions of the *Barefoot Doctor Handbook*—one published in Hunan Province is apparently widely available in China.[16] Excerpts from the table of contents of this book are shown in Appendix H. The diseases listed do not necessarily reflect their incidence and prevalence. Rickets, for example, was a highly prevalent disease in the past and is discussed in the handbook, but we were told that, with the improvement in dietary conditions and the availability of Vitamin D, rickets has been almost entirely eliminated. The only exception is in some areas of the northeast where sunshine, which produces Vitamin D in the body, is rare.

Another perhaps more direct measure of the barefoot doctor's role is the contents of his medical bag. In it are medications ranging from traditional herbs through drugs similar to our over-the-counter varieties such as aspirin and antacids, and to many of our prescription drugs such as penicillin and chlorpromazine. The bag also contains such items as alcohol, gentian violet, bandages, forceps, syringes, clinical thermometers, and acupuncture needles.

A standard list of the contents of the barefoot doctor's bag, provided by the Chinese Medical Association, is shown in Appendix G; indicated are those items we ourselves found in a barefoot doctor's bag in a commune near Shanghai. A careful review of these items with the barefoot doctor, as with the worker doctor, revealed a remarkably detailed knowledge on their part of the nature of the medications they dispensed, the indications and contraindications for their use, and their potential for causing adverse reactions.

Unfortunately there was insufficient opportunity to observe the activities of any barefoot doctor over a long period of time, and it is therefore impossible to comment on the "quality" of care being delivered; the observations we were able to make, however, suggest that care seems to be easily accessible and appropriate to the level of the problems presented, and that consultation and referral for more specialized clinical cases appear to be available. The barefoot doctor may be neither barefoot nor a doctor, but his fellow workers know him well and trust him.

HEALTH FACILITIES AT THE BRIGADE LEVEL

While facilities for health care at the brigade level vary widely in communes throughout China, the Sing Sing Production Brigade health center is fairly typical of those we visited. It is a one-room building furnished with a table, chairs, an examining table, and a medicine cabinet stocked with traditional and Western medicines. Here, in the fields, and in the patients' homes four barefoot doctors care for the brigade members.

The Tachai Brigade, famous throughout China for the near-miraculous way it transformed the once brown and barren hillsides of Shansi Province into green, flourishing farmland, in spite of natural disasters and with little help from the central government, has a far more elaborate health center. The Tachai Brigade clinic, although situated on the brigade's land, actually serves the entire commune of which the brigade is a unit. Housed in what was once a landlord's manor atop one of the hills of Tachai, it might more properly be described as a small commune hospital.

Thirteen medical workers operate out of the clinic: one

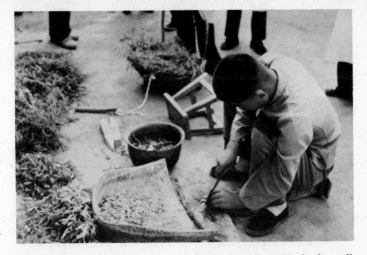

Barefoot doctor, Tachai Brigade health station, chopping herb medicines.

cadre, three doctors, three assistant doctors, who, as often happened, were identified to us as "doctors," two pharmacists, two nurse-midwives, one laboratory technician, and one dental technician. The three regular doctors were graduates of the medical school in the nearby provincial capital, Taiyuan. Of the three assistant doctors, two had attended middle medical schools and one had been "trained in the countryside." Dr. Liu Chi, a regularly trained city doctor who showed us the clinic, has lived and worked in the rural areas for ten years.

The clinic has trained thirty-three barefoot doctors to treat the 10,000 members of the twenty-one brigades that comprise the Tachai Commune. The barefoot doctors received one year of training on a half-time basis in a work-study program, a pattern different from that of the other communes we visited. They return to the clinic for further training when there is little work to be done in the fields.

Of the thirty-three, thirteen are women who were also trained in family planning and midwifery. As in other communes, normal deliveries are made at home; complicated cases are sent to the clinic to be attended by a nurse-midwife. Abortions, tubal ligations, and vas deferens ligations are also performed in the clinic.

Dr. Liu reported few cases of heart disease or cancer among the commune's population, and a "low rate of death under the age of sixty." After the age of sixty, people tend to die of lung disease, including tuberculosis, and cerebrovascular disease.

The clinic, in which approximately 200 minor operations had been performed during the first nine months of 1972, has a 50 kv. machine that is used for taking X-rays of chests and fractured limbs. The clinic also has facilities for distilling water and a sterilizer, and produces its own glucose solutions and normal saline. Clinic workers themselves prepare some of the herb medicines they use.

In contrast to the simple yet sturdy health center at the Sing Sing Production Brigade, and the elaborate clinic-hospital at the Tachai Brigade, the health station of the Shuan Wang Production Brigade of the Shuan Wang Commune outside of Sian is constructed of wooden planks and straw. A straw mat hanging over the opening serves as a door. The walls are made of smooth, dried mud, as are all the brigade's houses, and the dirt floor is trodden flat. Straw matting placed across two wooden boards serves as the examining table. Three barefoot doctors and seven health workers, one for each production team, staff the health station. The barefoot doctors rotate, with one always on duty in the health station while the other two visit the production teams or do agricultural work. The health workers are primarily responsible for immunizations and educating the women of the brigade about birth control.

COMMUNE HOSPITALS

Many large communes have their own hospital facilities to which patients are referred from the production brigade health stations. In the ten counties that comprise the Shanghai municipality there are 212 commune hospitals, each with an average of thirty beds. The Ma Chiao (Horse Bridge) Commune outside Shanghai, for example, has a thirty-bed hospital for a population of 35,000.

The China-Rumania Friendship People's Commune in the suburbs southwest of Peking also has a thirty-bed hospital, opened on May 10, 1971, to serve the 46,000 commune residents. The staff of fifty-nine includes twenty-five barefoot doctors, five Western-trained and two traditional doctors, and fifteen nurses, as well as technicians, administrators, and a cook. The hospital has no cleaning staff; all the staff help with the cleaning.

When we visited the hospital in the fall of 1972, 8,000 people had been treated on an outpatient and 500 on an inpatient basis since the hospital opened. The hospital has thirteen "departments": surgery, ENT, internal medicine, traditional medicine, "women's," public health, radiology, laboratory, emergency, inpatient, pharmacy (that dispenses both Western and traditional medicines), a factory that produces medicines, and a supply service.

We were told by Yin Shih-chie, chairman of the hospital's revolutionary committee, that it costs 70,000 *yüan* (U.S.$28,000) a year to operate the hospital—30,000 *yüan* for wages and 40,000 for medical equipment. The funds are raised in part from the 5 *fen* registration fee all patients pay, and from the higher fees charged to the 5 per cent of the commune population who are not permitted to join its cooperative health system—former landlords, "reactionaries," and "right-wing elements," who are considered "class enemies." The remainder of the funds is contributed by the commune. The doctors, all of whom are on a one-year rotation from the Fenghei District Hospital in Peking, earn from 42 to 79.50 *yüan* a month; nurses' salaries range from 42 to 56.50. The doctors, we were told, work in the fields one day a week.

The medical personnel in the public health department consist of a barefoot doctor, a nurse, and a middle medical doctor who graduated in 1962 from a three-year course at Peking Medical College. They reported to us the following incidence of infectious diseases in the commune from January through August 1972:

	Cases	Per 1,000 Population Annually
Measles	35	1.2
Diarrhea	340	11.0
Hepatitis	100	4.0
Tuberculosis	345	11.0
Pertussis	4	0.1

There were no reported cases of encephalitis, meningitis, diphtheria, poliomyelitis, or tetanus.

The public health department also cooperates on a family planning program with the women's department and with the brigade's barefoot doctors. The staff told us that there are 5,777 married women of "childbearing age" in the commune. The number using each type of contraceptive is shown in Table 8. Of the remaining women not using birth control, they said, "some have just gotten married," and "some have only one child." In 1971 some 1,181 babies were born on the China-Rumania Friendship People's Commune, for a birth rate of 26 per 1,000, a remarkable reduction from the former rate, which may have been on the order of 45 per 1,000. While it is considerably lower than

TABLE 8. BIRTH CONTROL FIGURES FOR THE CHINA-RUMANIA PEOPLE'S FRIENDSHIP COMMUNE, 1972

		Per cent		Per cent
Total number of commune members	46,000	100		
Married women of childbearing age	5,777	12		100
Women using pill			1,323	23
Women using IUD			1,035	18
Husbands using condom			526	9
Total using contraception			2,884	50
Women who have had tubal ligations			458	8
Husbands who have had vasectomies			126	2
Total sterilized			584	10

the rate in the past, the commune leaders would like to lower it to 15 per 1,000.

In the internal medicine department two doctors work together—a male graduate of a medical college in northeast China and a female barefoot doctor. They see thirty to forty patients a day, each treating a different patient, working side-by-side in the same room. If the barefoot doctor, who has been working at this hospital for two years, has questions she discusses them with her coworker.

The department of traditional Chinese medicine treats approximately 120 patients daily, most of whom are self-referred. Pulse diagnosis is used, and treatment includes acupuncture and herbal medicines. A patient being seen during our visit was complaining of abdominal pain she had had for several hours. After a barefoot doctor had examined her and noted her symptoms, a combination of traditional Chinese and Western medicines were prescribed. When we asked what course would be taken if there had been a suspicion of appendicitis, the traditional doctor in charge replied that if there were evidence of acute appendicitis the patient would be referred to the surgical department; if the pain was chronic, however, she would be treated with traditional Chinese medicine and acupuncture.

The Shuan Wang People's Commune in Shensi Province is thirty-five miles east of Sian in Weinan county, which has a population of 400,000. The commune's population of 15,600 has a new, red brick hospital whose director is Han Chu-ying, a modest, gentle-looking, young female middle medical school graduate. Dr. Han, who had earlier lived in the countryside, entered Pao Chi Medical School in 1963 but did not complete the four-year course until 1968 because the onset of the Cultural Revolution delayed classes for a year. After graduation Dr. Han worked in another commune until 1971, when the Bureau of Public Health of Weinan County appointed her director of this commune hospital. In addition to her duties as director, Dr. Han practices internal medicine.

Ten regular and middle medical doctors, including Dr. Han, one nurse, two pharmacists, and a cook work at the hospital.

Two doctors are graduates of higher medical school, four, including one trained in traditional medicine, of middle medical school, and four, including two trained in traditional medicine, had predominantly practical training, with only a short period of formal education. The two doctors with regular training are surgeons—a man who is permanently assigned to the hospital and a woman on rotation from Sian Medical College.

Although the hospital had no inpatient beds as of September 1972—they plan to have forty eventually—four to five fairly major operations are performed each month, and one room is available for postoperative surgical patients. The staff also performs abortions, using an electric suction machine, difficult deliveries, and appendectomies, and inserts intrauterine devices.

The doctors go to higher-level hospitals for further training on a rotating basis while continuing to receive full salary. Just prior to our visit one of the physicians had spent six weeks in the county hospital receiving further gynecological training. Thirty-three barefoot doctors from the commune were trained in the same county hospital, and they in turn have trained 128 health workers.

County Hospitals

In 1965, before the onset of the Cultural Revolution, Chang Tze-k'uan of the Department of Medical Administration of the Chinese Ministry of Health wrote in the *Chinese Medical Journal:*

> . . . Today, every one of China's 2,000 or so counties has a fairly well equipped and competently staffed general hospital. Most of these county hospitals have about 100 beds and the larger ones have from 200 to 300 beds. In recent years large numbers of graduates from colleges and schools of medicine and pharmaceutics have been assigned to work in county hospitals, and in many regions senior physicians have been transferred from city hospitals to county hospitals to add strength to rural health work.[17]

County hospitals are generally located in the towns and serve the people of the area as well as patients referred from the commune hospitals. The hospital for Shunyi County, a part of the Peking municipality northeast of the city proper, has a staff of 104 men and 114 women to run its ambulatory and inpatient services for the 450,000 members of the nineteen communes in the county. Of this staff, 143 are medical workers—forty-eight doctors, sixty-three nurses, and thirty-two pharmacists and technicians. In addition to this hospital, seven commune hospitals and twelve commune clinics provide medical care in the county. In all, 676 medical workers (excluding barefoot doctors and health workers) serve the population of Shunyi County: 312 doctors, sixty-five nurses, and 299 pharmacists and technicians.

The chairman of the revolutionary committee of the county hospital, Wang Chan-hao, a cadre not a doctor, told us the committee is made up of eleven members, five full-time and six part-time, eight men and three women. The full-time members are the chairman, three vice-chairmen in charge of professional work, administration, and public health, respectively, and one leading member in charge of administration. The six part-time members are doctors, nurses, and workers in the hospital. While only hospital staff belong to the committee, the members do "listen to the opinions of the poor and lower-middle peasants and workers" when planning the medical work of the hospital.

Funds for the hospital come from the financial department of the county. Comrade Wang told us that the revolutionary committee prepares the annual budget, which must finally be approved by the municipality of which Shunyi County is a part. He stated that the hospital usually receives the funds requested.

The county hospital demonstrates the same concern with birth control as is seen at the brigade and commune levels. Table 9 shows the types of contraception and sterilization being used in the county; contraception methods include a monthly, injected hormone preparation that has been used since 1970. The 20,000 women who are not using birth control are either "newly married, ill, or have only daughters, no sons thus far." As a result of these efforts only 9,504 babies were born in Shunyi County in 1971, a rate of 21 per 1,000 population. Although this is already a low rate in comparison with other rural areas, as in the other regions the hope is to lower it to 15 per 1,000 by 1975.

After a normal delivery the mothers remain in the hospital for three to five days at a total cost of 10 *yüan*. Opening off the

TABLE 9. BIRTH CONTROL FIGURES FOR SHUNYI COUNTY, PEKING

		Per cent		Per cent
Total population	450,000	100		
Total married women of child-bearing age	49,297	11		100
Women using pill			10,000	20
Women receiving monthly contraceptive injections			515	1
Women using the IUD			14,151	29
Couples using rhythm			2,300	5
Couples using barriers (diaphragm or condom)			1,004	2
Total using contraceptives			27,970	57
Women who have had tubal ligations			1,596	3
Husbands who have had vasectomies			281	0.6
Total sterilized			1,877	4

dark corridors of the hospital, the nursery is bright and clean. Only one-third of the tiny cribs were filled with sleeping babies wrapped up to their necks in blankets with their arms firmly tucked under the blankets. (The nursery staff complained to us of the shortage of babies due to the success of birth control efforts.)

The children's ward was darkened to enable the patients to sleep. The mothers of almost every child were by their bedside, particularly the more severely ill children. The doctors told us that mothers are permitted to stay with their children all night if their condition is serious.

The clinics of the Shunyi County Hospital had 162,996 patient-visits from January to August 1972, an average of 668 daily. During the same period, 3,474 inpatients were treated for a total of 36,032 inpatient days. The average patient stay is ten days, and an average of 147 patients occupy the 155 hospital beds on any given day (95 percent average occupancy). Of the 130 patients who died in the hospital between January and August, autopsies were done on only four.

PAYMENT FOR MEDICAL CARE

As in the cities, methods of payment for medical care in the communes vary widely. Peasants in many communes may participate in a collective medical care system, each family paying into the fund an annual premium for each of its members. The entire family is then covered for all medical expenses except for payment of a nominal registration fee. In the Mai Chia Wu Production Brigade of the West Lake People's Commune outside Hangchow, for example, a premium of 1 yüan (U.S. 40 cents) is paid annually for each person, including children, and all medical expenses, including hospitalization, are paid by the cooperative.

The Shuan Wang Production Brigade near Sian also has a cooperative medical system under which each peasant pays 50 fen (U.S. 20 cents) a year into the fund; the brigade's public welfare fund contributes an equal amount. Patients must still pay a 5 fen registration fee each time they see a doctor, however, and, as is the custom in China, hospitalized patients pay for their food.

The Tachai Brigade, on the other hand, has quite a different system of payment for medical care. They use what Dr. Liu Chi calls the "three point system": (1) If a patient's illness is work-related, all medical care is free; (2) if he is seriously ill and cannot afford medical care, the brigade helps with the payment; and (3) if he has a "light disease" and can pay for treatment, he does so.

In any event payment is minimal at the Tachai clinic. There is no registration fee, nor any charge for injections, acupuncture treatments, or home visits. If a patient with a cold is treated with acupuncture there is no charge; if medicine is prescribed he "pays a few fen." Dr. Liu contrasted the cost of medicine in 1949 to the present cost; after Liberation one penicillin capsule cost 1 yüan; it costs now 10 percent of that—10 fen.

When we asked Dr. Liu why the brigade did not have a cooperative medical system as do other brigades, and thus remove the burden of medical payments, he replied that the income of brigade members has increased rapidly: "Every working day each worker earns approximately 1.5 yüan; 95 per cent of the brigade's families earn enough so they have savings and can afford to pay directly for their medical care. Therefore, the brigade has not considered changing the system."

Thus, just as the training of barefoot doctors, the physical characteristics of the brigade health stations, and the facilities available at the commune level vary throughout China, so too does payment for medical care. But within these variations, and within regional characteristics and the different economic levels of the communes, at least a minimum standard of health care now seems available to all of China's peasants.

Notes

1. *1970 Census of Population PC (VI)-1 United States* (Washington, D.C.: Bureau of the Census, 1971).

2. *Narodnoe Khoziaistovo SSSR v 1968 Godu (People's Economy, USSR, 1968)* (Moscow: Central Statistical Unit, 1969): p. 7.

3. Morris Harth, ed., *The New York Times Encyclopedic Almanac 1971* (New York: New York Times, 1972): p. 715.

4. William Hinton, *Fanshen: A Documentary of Revolution in a Chinese Village* (New York: Vantage Press [Random House], 1966).

5. John B. Grant, "Rural Reconstruction in China," in *Health Care for the Community: Selected Papers of Dr. John B. Grant*, ed., Conrad Seipp (Baltimore: Johns Hopkins Press, 1963): pp. 148-54.

6. Report of an Investigation from Shanghai, "The Orientation of the Revolution in Medical Education as Seen in the Growth of 'Barefoot Doctors'," *China's Medicine* no. 10 (October 1968): 574-81.

7. John A.D. Cooper, "Education for the Health Professions in the Soviet Union," *Journal of Medical Education* 46 (1971): 412-18.

8. Patrick B. Storey, *"The Soviet Feldsher as a Physician's Assistant* (Washington, D.C.: Department of Health, Education, and Welfare Publication No. (NIH) 72-58, February, 1972).

9. "Everybody Works for Good Health," *China Reconstructs* 10 (November 1971): 20-22.

10. Joshua S. Horn, *Away with All Pests . . . An English Surgeon in People's China* (New York: Monthly Review Press, 1971): pp. 135-40.

11. Victor W. Sidel, "Feldshers and 'Feldsherism'," *New England Journal of Medicine* 278 (1968): 939-40, 981-92.

12. ———, "The Feldsher in the U.S.S.R.," *Annals of the New York Academy of Sciences* 166 (1969): 957-66.

13. G. A Kovrigin and A. Matlin, "Glavnoe v nashem dele—seno" ("The Greatest of Our Concerns—Hay: Story of a Village Feldsher"), *Krokodil* (August 24, 1968): 10-11.

14. E. F. Rosinski and F. J. Spencer, *The Assistant Medical Officer* (Chapel Hill: University of North Carolina Press, 1965).

15. N.R.E. Fendall, *Auxiliaries in Health Care* (Baltimore: Johns Hopkins Press for the Josiah Macy, Jr. Foundation, 1972).

16. Hunan Chinese Medical and Pharmaceutical Institute Revolutionary Committee, *Chijiao Yisheng Shouce (Barefoot Doctor Handbook)* (Hunan: People's Publishers, 1970).

17. Chang Tze-K'uan, "The Development of Hospital Service in China," *Chinese Medical Journal* 84 (1965): 412-16.

IV. The Role of the Community and the Patient in Health Care

PRIOR to the founding of the Republic in 1912, there is little evidence of any systematic attempt to involve the individual or the community in an active role in health care or in the prevention of illness. During the epidemics which struck Imperial China so disasterously, recourse was often made to magic rather than to public health practice. According to Huard and Wong, "During the plague epidemic which struck Mengtsz in 1896 the *taotai* assembled the soldiers of his guard each evening in front of his *yamen* and made them give salvoes in all directions to frighten the demon of the plague." [1]

Free vaccinations were first begun in China in 1903, but lack of understanding of their value and superstition delayed their maximum use. By 1928, however, 500,000 free vaccinations had been given,[2] and in the late 1920s and early 1930s mass campaigns were held in Canton against smallpox and in Shanghai against cholera. These efforts were accompanied by health education campaigns carried out initially by the YMCA and the YWCA.[3] Health surveys, health campaigns, and the distribution of health literature were later conducted by both national and local governments. In Szechwan the West China Council on Health Education, started by missionary doctors, sponsored a program which included the distribution of health materials, including posters and books, to schools, and smallpox eradication campaigns.[4]

But, as Ralph Croizier has so aptly stated, "For its net effect on health conditions in China as a whole, all of this, like the Republic itself, was little more than a declaration of intent." [5] It was left to the Communist government to mobilize and educate the Chinese people with respect to their massive health problems.

POST-LIBERATION PRINCIPLES AND PRACTICE

Mao Tse-tung in his essay *On Practice* in 1937 wrote:

> If you want to know the taste of a pear, you must change the pear by eating it yourself. If you want to know the structure and properties of the atom, you must make physical and chemical experiments to change the state of the atom. If you want to know the theory and methods of revolution, you must take part in revolution. All genuine knowledge originates in direct experience.[6]

This theme of knowing by doing runs through essentially all aspects of Chinese life today. A peasant learns the difficulties of determining agricultural priorities by taking part in decision-making. The urban doctor learns about the life of the peasants by moving to the countryside for a period of time and laboring with them. The child learns what it is like to be a peasant or a worker by growing vegetables or doing a job on consignment from a factory. And, according to this theory, the way to teach 800 million people the principles of health prevention and health care is to involve them in it.

The mobilization of the mass has been the primary technique by which the Chinese have accomplished their feats of engineering: the construction of their canals, bridges, large-scale irrigation projects, and dikes, and the damming of rivers. The mobilization of the mass has been the key mechanism in their feats of human engineering also. Han Suyin describes the process of education of the masses since 1949 as one that has included the "eradication of the feudal mind," and "getting the masses away from the anchored belief that natural calamities are 'fixed by heaven' and that therefore nothing can be done to remedy one's lot . . ." She continues: "To bridge this gap between scientific modern man and feudal man, the prey of superstition, and to do it within the compass of one generation, is a formidible task."[7] One important technique used to accomplish this "formidible task" has been the activating of the mass. In health care this has meant the broadest involvement of people at every level of society in movements such as the Patriotic Health Campaign; the recruitment of selected groups of people such as barefoot doctors from the population they are to serve; and the mobilization of the individual to "fight against his own disease." Individual concern with health reflects the Chinese belief in *tzu-li keng-sheng*, or self-reliance, more accurately translated as "regeneration through one's own efforts"—a virtue as honored today as its converse, mutual help.

This was brought home to us most strikingly while we were observing a kindergarten class of six-year-olds. They were being taught the life story of Norman Bethune, a Canadian thoracic surgeon who provided medical services for Mao Tse-tung's Eighth Route Army in the war against Japan until his death in 1939 from septicemia, secondary to an infection he acquired while performing surgery. Dr. Bethune is a national hero in China, celebrated for his "selflessness," his internationalism, and his self-reliance—all principles that are taught to Chinese children. After the audiovisual presentation the children were asked what they would do if they came upon a sick person on the street. "I would get water for him," and "I would get medicine for him," were typical replies, all suggesting things the child himself could do for the sick man rather than going to get help from a doctor or other adult.

THE ROLE OF THE MASS

In the early 1950s, in conjunction with the fourth of Mao's Four Main Health Principles, "Health work should be combined with the mass movement," the Patriotic Health Campaign was launched. Horn states that the Chinese linked the campaign to the need to protect the population against the alleged use of germ warfare by the United States in Korea; [8] the Chinese with whom we spoke, however, never mentioned germ warfare. The primary goal of the mass movement in the early fifties, we were told, was the elimination of mosquitoes, flies, rats, and sparrows, and the people were mobilized to exterminate these pests under the guidance of health personnel. The Patriotic Health Campaign has been maintained and has been expanded to include the sanitary aspects of food, water, and the environment.

While environmental sanitation is a constant activity, it is attacked with particular intensity around festival days and in preparation for the May 1 and October 1 celebrations. Everyone participates, from retired people to health activists, and the general population works under the leadership of medical personnel. Thursday morning, we were told during our 1971 visit to Shanghai, is the fixed time for cleaning: the people scour the streets and their homes; cadres who work in the government usually do manual labor one day a week, often on cleanup day. There is interdistrict inspection whereby a group of people from one district come in and inspect another area and criticize or exchange experiences. We were told by Dr. Hong Ming-gui, leading member of the Shanghai branch of the Chinese Medical Association, that criticism most often takes the form of "promoting the strong points of another district, encouraging that district." He also quoted the slogan used around cleanup time: "It's a glorious thing to speak about hygiene and you should be ashamed if you're very dirty." (One assumes this sounds somewhat different in Chinese.) Dr. Hong stressed the importance of the involvement of the masses in breaking with traditional habits and in changing the spirit of the people.

Health workers in a neighborhood health station in Hangchow, which serves 28,000 people, told us that they have established three days a month as general cleanup days. The entire population is mobilized into groups, and certain individuals in each group are responsible for wiping out the pests, eliminating their breeding places, disinfecting water, and keeping the neighborhood clean.

This health station uses more than 100 different herbs to treat chronic diseases, and people in the neighborhood climb a nearby mountain to plant and gather herbs; they are also educated as to their use.

"Health propaganda," as the Chinese put it, plays a crucial role in the participation of the community in health problems. Great attention is paid to educating the populace on the importance of immunizations, the handling of infectious diseases, and the need for "planned birth."

In a district general hospital in Peking we were told of both mass meetings and study groups in the twenty-three neighborhood health stations under its jurisdiction; the meetings are organized by the health workers in the district to educate the people in hygiene and in the prevention of infectious disease, which they are taught to report to the health center immediately. These meetings are conducted on a regular basis as well as at special times during the year. The health station itself is considered a "mass organization."

On one wall of the hospital was a list of responsibilities of the Red Medical Workers (see Table 4, page 54). Responsibility No. 3 states that stress should be put on prevention and on the patriotic hygiene movement, with a general cleaning every week and a thorough general cleaning every two weeks, and on propaganda on how to deal with infectious disease, vaccinations, and combining treatment and prevention.

Orleans and Suttemeier [9] have emphasized the importance in China of mobilizing the masses in dealing with the problem of pollution. They describe people organized in the cities to "remove refuse that had accumulated in a residential district" and, more specifically, "the spring patriotic sanitation movement" of 1970 that was organized by local revolutionary committees to mobilize the people to pick up litter and garbage from residences, farms, and factories, to clean up local water supplies, to eliminate pests, to collect reusable wastes, and to advocate public health measures. They also describe the efforts of the Shanghai Municipal Revolutionary Committee in July 1968 to clean up the Whangpoo River and Soochow Creek. The authors quote the *New China News Agency* as stating that

> . . . 90,000 persons were mobilized on the industrial and agricultural fronts in Shanghai to form muck-dredging and muck-transporting teams, waging a vehement people's war to dredge muck from the Suchow River [sic]. After 100 days of turbulent fighting, more than 403,600 tons of maladorous organic mire had been dug out.

The classic example of the use of mass organization in health has, of course, been the campaign against schistosomiasis. According to Horn this campaign was based on the concept of the "mass line"—"the conviction that the ordinary people possess great

strength and wisdom and that when their initiative is given full
play they can accomplish miracles." [10] Before the peasants were
organized to fight against the snails, Horn states, they were
thoroughly educated in the nature of schistosomiasis by means of
lectures, films, posters, and radio talks. They were then mobilized
twice a year, in March and in August, and, along with voluntary
labor from the People's Liberation Army, students, teachers, and
office workers, they drained the rivers and ditches, buried the
banks of the rivers, and smoothed down the buried dirt. Horn
points out that in the antischistosomiasis program the concept
was not only to recruit the mass to do the work but to mobilize
their enthusiasm and initiative so that they would fight the
disease.[11]

This method of attacking the enemy is an adaptation by
Mao of the successful methods used in wartime Yenan to fire
the enthusiasm of the population against the Japanese. Mao has
transferred this ideology into campaigns against such "enemies"
as illiteracy, disease, famine, and flood. In this case the enemy is
schistosomiasis, and the technique used is the well-known "paper
tiger" theory first used by Mao in 1946 to describe the United
States–Kuomintang alliance. It states that there is a dual nature
to everything—while one's enemies are real and formidible and
must be taken seriously, they are at the same time paper tigers
that can be defeated by the will of the people. One has to view
one's enemies from this dual point of view, Mao teaches, in order
to plan correctly one's strategy and one's tactics.

The antischistosomiasis effort is particularly revealing, since
it mobilized the population in several directions: to move against
the snails, to cooperate in case finding and treatment, and to
improve environmental sanitation. Yukiang County in Kiangsi
Province, for example, had been plagued by schistosomiasis for
more than 100 years. According to one report, 1 million m.^{2} of
land was infested with snails, and the "average" infection rate
among the peasants was 21.4 per cent.[12] After investigating the
prevalence of the disease, an antischistosomiasis station was set up
in the county in 1953. When the campaign started, the personnel
of the station began publicizing its purpose, as well as health work

in general, using ". . . broadcasting, wall newspapers, black-boards, exhibits of real and model objects, lantern-slide shows, and dramatic performances. Related scientific knowledge was also popularized. To help the peasants raise their political conscious-ness, break their superstitious belief in gods, devils, and fate, and to build up their confidence in conquering the disease, meetings were organized for recalling sufferings in the old society and comparing them with the happiness in the new society. Through these activities the confidence of the broad mass in the certain triumph of their struggle against schistosomiasis was gradually built up and further strengthened." [13]

Once the population learned about schistosomiasis, a "peo-ple's war" was launched against the snails. From 1955 to 1957, 20,000 peasants in Yukiang County filled up old ditches and ponds, dug new ditches, and expanded the cultivation area by roughly ninety acres. Special methods had to be used in some areas. For example, three three-feet-deep lotus ponds covering several acres had a high density of snails that people had attempted to exterminate by removing the surface soil, by burning aquatic vegetation, and by other methods, but the snails had not been completely eliminated. Finally the ponds were drained, all grass and vegetation at the bottom were burned, and snail-free mud was piled on top and pounded so that the snails were suffocated. Seven square or rectangular fish ponds were then created out of the three former snail-breeding ponds. [14]

After this massive war on schistosomiasis, however, it was still necessary to check for the recurrence of snails, as well as on water control and waste disposal, so the people had to be educated in the treatment of human excreta, the provision of safe drinking water, and improved personal hygiene. Production teams under the leadership of health workers are responsible for these public health measures.

Horn reports the need to instruct the population on the importance of regular feces examination. At one commune he was told that the peasants did not always take the testing seri-ously and tried to play jokes on the testers by substituting dog or ox dung. The testers met this problem by reminding the peasants

of what life had been like in the "bitter past" when schistosomiasis was common; cooperation was soon restored.[15]

Health work in Heilungkiang Province in the northeast
was cited in an article in *China's Medicine* in 1968.[16] In order to
spread health education in the province, mass meetings were called
in sixty cities and counties, leaflets and pamphlets on health were
distributed, and students then began to engage in health education among the workers and peasants. It was estimated that in
two counties 250,000 middle and primary school students were
mobilized for this work. Needless to say, the students learned
as much as they taught.

The Role of Indigenous Health Personnel

Since the Cultural Revolution it has been common practice
in both urban neighborhoods and the communes to recruit health
personnel from among the indigenous population. The barefoot
doctors in the countryside, the Red Medical Workers in the cities,
the worker doctors in the factories, and the health workers in the
cities and on the communes are members of the mass recruited
to provide health care and to communicate what they have
learned to their friends and neighbors. In Silvery Lane in
Hangchow, a community of 702 families, fifty residents work in
the health center in official capacities; in other words, one member
out of every fourteen families in the lane is directly responsible
for health care. The high percentage of residents in any given
neighborhood who are active in health work are responsible for
instructing the rest of the community in the need for immunizations, the use of birth control, and the importance of good sanitation. We were astounded at the high rate of immunizations in the
Peking health station we visited (see Chapter II). It became clear
that because of the closely-knit neighborhood, and the integration
of the health station with the neighborhood, few children go
unattended.

This is also true in the Hangchow health center, where the
personnel keep track of the contraception method each family
is using by visiting each home once a month. When we asked if
the women were reluctant to discuss their methods of contraception we were told that occasionally a newly married woman

might be shy, but that once the importance of birth control to China is explained, she cooperates. The large number of health workers and their commitment to health propaganda combine to make each contact a health education contact.

The commune health workers receive neither extra pay nor time off from their regular jobs. They do their health work during their lunch periods or at the end of the day. In addition to treating minor illnesses and giving immunizations, these individuals are responsible for disinfecting the water and treating human feces (night soil), which is used as fertilizer. These health workers are trained by, and are under the supervision of, the barefoot doctors.

The elimination of venereal disease in China provides another example of both the mobilization and education of the people and the use of indigenous health personnel. As Felix Greene describes it, people were organized around the slogan: "We don't want to take syphilis into Communism." In the early 1950's checklists of symptoms were posted in every store and every community center throughout the country, and anyone with any of the symptoms was urged to get a blood test and be treated. Neighborhood pressure was brought to bear on those who tended to ignore symptoms or who had a history of promiscuity. Where the concentration of the disease was great, specially trained individuals in the neighborhoods made door-to-door visits to give examinations and blood tests. Prostitutes were identified, and suitable alternative jobs were found for them—if necessary by moving equipment, such as sewing machines, into the brothels and turning them into factories. Thus, prostitution was outlawed. Neighborhood committees had, and continue to have, the authority to eliminate prostitution and promiscuity. The technical details of the conquest of venereal disease are described in Edgar Snow's biographical chapter on Dr. Ma Hai-teh,[17] and in Ma's own article on the subject in *China's Medicine* in 1966.[18]

THE ROLE OF THE PATIENT

The third way in which the Chinese people are encouraged to be involved in health is through mobilization of the individual patient. In the psychiatric ward of the Peking Third Hospital we were told that the staff tries to "promote the active factors so that the patient can struggle against his own disease." The patient studies the works of Chairman Mao in order to understand his illness and to be able to fight against it. As the psychiatrists told us, "Through the patient's studies, his ideology is much elevated. The patient can then investigate his disease and recognize his condition in order to prevent a relapse." The following description of his illness was given us by a thirty-eight-year-old male patient in the psychiatric ward of the Peking Third Hospital:

> My main trouble is suspicion. I think my ceiling is going to fall down; when big character posters are up I think it is criticism of myself; and when somebody is gossiping I think they are talking about me.
>
> After I was admitted to this hospital I gradually recognized my illness. As Chairman Mao says, when we face a problem we have to face it thoroughly, not only from one side. When I am discharged from the hospital, the doctors have said that I should have some problem of investigation in my mind. When I am in touch with people they have suggested that I make conclusions in my mind after investigation not before investigation, in order to see if what I suspect to be true is just subjective thinking or is objectively correct. By studying Chairman Mao we can treat and cure disease.

The Shanghai Mental Hospital has carried the idea of a patient's disease as his enemy a step further. They have "adopted the system used in the army" and have divided the staff of the hospital into four divisions. The patients on the wards have also been divided into groups, and they now comprise a "collective fighting group instead of a ward." One of the psychiatrists told us, "It is not enough to have the doctors' or nurses' initiative; we need the patients' initiative to work together against the disease." This view of the patient's relationship with his mental illness is a curious combination of individual responsibility and viewing the illness as an external enemy, a dual attitude that perhaps serves to maximize the patient's efforts to fight his illness, while leaving him less guilt-ridden if he fails.

Patients are not only expected to participate in their own care; they are also expected to help one another. The Shanghai

Mental Hospital has a buddy system whereby the healthier patients who have been in the hospital longer help the newer, sicker patients to adjust to their surroundings and to understand their illness.

Horn describes a patient whose burns covered 89 per cent of the surface of his body. At one point during treatment the patient's appetite started to diminish and, as days went on, he ate less and less. The dietitian tried to tempt him with delicacies, and chefs in Shanghai restaurants produced special menus to encourage him to eat; but, most important, "his comrades urged him to eat as a political duty, as his contribution to the fight for his life that was being waged with such determination by so many." [19]

In an article entitled "How We Have Struggled against Unstable Diabetes Mellitus in the Light of Mao Tse-tung's Thought," [20] three patients write of their difficulties in dealing with their diabetes over the years and of the new approach they took in managing their disease: they studied the "pathophysiology of diabetes," "became familiar with the regulation of insulin dosage," and applied the theory of the paper tiger, that is, "we despised him and we took him seriously." Thus, the article states, the patients' initiative to fight against their diabetes was mobilized and their disease stabilized.

In health, as in other aspects of the Chinese brand of social-ism, there are no passive bystanders. One is expected to participate "wholeheartedly" in community public health measures, in the organization of medical care, and in the conduct of all aspects of one's personal life, including one's health. It is a country of mass and individual participation, of mass and individual responsi-bility. John G. Gurley, an economist, has described China's cur-rent view of the role of the people in the following way:

> To gain knowledge, people must be awakened from their half slumber, encouraged to mobilize themselves and to take conscious action to elevate and liberate themselves. When they actively par-ticipate in decision-making, when they take an interest in state affairs, when they dare to do new things, when they become good at presenting facts and reasoning things out, when they criticize

and test and experiment scientifically, having discarded myths and superstitions, when they are aroused—then the socialist initiative latent in the masses [will] burst out with volcanic force.[21]

In stressing participation and mutual responsibility, the Chinese over the past twenty-four years have accomplished astonishing feats in the field of medicine and public health, and have educated their enormous population to an increased awareness and understanding of preventive medicine and medical care. For the Chinese do believe, as Mao teaches, that: "If you want knowledge, you must take part in the practice of changing reality." [22]

NOTES

1. Pierre Huard and Ming Wong, *Chinese Medicine* (London: World University Library, 1968): p. 70.

2. Herbert Day Lamson, *Social Pathology in China* (Shanghai: The Commercial Press, 1935): p. 457.

3. Ibid., p. 458.

4. Ibid., pp. 483-84.

5. Ralph C. Croizier, *Traditional Medicine in Modern China* (Cambridge: Harvard University Press, 1968): p. 47.

6. Mao Tse-tung, "On Practice," *Four Essays on Philosophy* (Peking: Foreign Languages Press, 1966): p. 8.

7. Han Suyin, "Reflections on Social Change," *Bulletin of the Atomic Scientists* 22, no. 6 (1966): 80-83.

8. Joshua S. Horn, *Away with All Pests . . . An English Surgeon in People's China.* (New York: Monthly Review Press, 1971): p. 126.

9. Leo A. Orleans and Richard P. Suttmeier, "The Mao Ethic and Environmental Quality," *Science* 170 (1970): 1173-76.

10. Horn, *Away with All Pests,* p. 96.

11. Ibid., p. 97.

12. "A Great Victory of Mao Tse-tung's Thought in the Battle against Schistosomiasis," *China's Medicine* 10 (October 1968): 588-602.

13. Ibid., p. 593.

14. Ibid., pp. 598-99.

15. Horn, *Away with All Pests,* p. 99.

16. "Experiences in Health Work and Disease Prevention in Heilungkiang Province in the Past Year," *China's Medicine* (March 1968): 148-53.

17. Edgar Snow, *Red China Today* (New York: Vintage Books, 1970): pp. 261-69.

18. George Hatem, "With Mao Tse-tung's Thought as the Compass for Action in the Control of Venereal Disease in China," *China's Medicine* 1 (October 1966): 52-67.

19. Horn, *Away with All Pests,* p. 108.

20. Chang Tze-han, Yang Teh-ching, and Tu Jui-fen, "How We Have Struggled against Unstable Diabetes Mellitus in the Light of Mao Tse-tung's Thought," *China's Medicine* 7 (July 1968): 400-407.

21. John G. Gurley, "Capitalist and Maoist Economic Development," in *America's Asia,* eds. Edward Freedman and Mark Selden (New York: Vintage Books, 1971): p. 336.

22. Mao, "On Practice," p. 8.

V. Medical Education

MEDICAL SCHOOLS: PRE- AND POST-LIBERATION

THE earliest medical schools in China were established by missionaries and supported by groups in the United States, Germany, France, and Great Britain. Among those conducted under United States auspices were the Lingnan Medical School, now the Chungshan (Dr. Sun Yat-sen) Medical College in Kwangchow; the Hsiang-ya (Hunan-Yale) Medical College sponsored by the Yale Foreign Missionary Society; and the Harvard Medical School of China in Shanghai.[1,2] Two major foreign institutions in Shanghai were St. John's, an American-sponsored school from which Dr. Hsu Chia-yu, our 1971 interpreter, graduated in 1949, and Aurora, a French-sponsored school whose aging hospital buildings are now the home of the Juichin Hospital which we visited in 1971. The Peking Union Medical College, probably the most famous, was founded and supported by the Rockefeller Foundation and the China Medical Board.[3]

Despite—or, as the Chinese suggest, perhaps in part because of—the efforts of missionary doctors and their organizations, both lay and religious, relatively few doctors of Western medicine were trained in pre-Liberation China. The limited medical education facilities, and the limited production of "scientific" doctors, followed Western models that seemed at the time, as well as in retrospect, inappropriate and inadequate to meet China's massive needs for medical manpower.

In attempting to increase the number of physicians, one of the first actions in the post-Liberation period was to increase the number of medical personnel being trained, for the most part following Soviet models. For example, after the Soviet pattern, many medical schools were split up into faculties of adult therapeutic medicine, pediatrics, public health, and stomatology.

111

In 1957, after a British delegation visited China, Theodore Fox, editor of *The Lancet,* was critical of the trends in medical education he had observed. He described, for example, the difficulty of dealing with an annual class of 400 to 600 students, and of shortening the curriculum:

> Lasting harm is done to a profession, and the people it serves, by introducing new members who have not had a proper basic training . . . Much useful work can be done by people without a good basic training, but they should not be called doctors. In China, I would say, entry to the over-crowded medical colleges should be further curtailed, and the need for more "pairs of hands" in medicine should be met by training more feldshers . . .[4]

In 1962 the Ministry of Health decided that the curriculum in all "regular" medical colleges "should gradually be prolonged to six years." [5]

Wilder Penfield's description of medical schools during his trip to China in 1962 summarizes the types and length of training at that time:

> One college calls for a curriculum of eight years—the Chinese Medical College in Peking (. . . housed in the beautiful buildings of the former Peking Union Medical College . . .). It is planned to train teachers and research workers. Each physician should have mastered two foreign languages before graduation from this College. Of the other medical colleges, one-third now provide a six-year curriculum and less than two-thirds, a five-year curriculum. A very few schools have a three-year course, which is intended to prepare men [sic] for the practical needs of factories, mines, and farms.[6]

During the period 1949 through 1965, using Soviet models, large numbers of "secondary" or "middle" medical schools were developed that accepted graduates of junior middle schools, the equivalent of our junior high schools, and offered courses of about three years' duration. These schools graduated assistant doctors, nurses, midwives, and other "middle medical workers." As with the "regular" doctors, however, these new medical workers became heavily concentrated in the urban areas, and there were still grossly inadequate numbers of health care personnel in the rural areas.

Changes Brought by the Cultural Revolution

Attitudes in medicine reflected many of the traditional Chinese values held prior to Liberation, which persisted to some degree into the 1950s and 1960s. Intellectual endeavor was felt to be superior to physical labor; urban professionals lived in a different world from the peasant in the countryside; and the intellectual and managerial elite were felt to be perpetuating themselves by their children's better early education and consequent easier access to universities and professional schools.

When students entered medical school, class differentiation continued. In 1968 the revolutionary committee of the Shanghai First Medical College wrote of medical education prior to 1966:

. . . Under its decayed system and time-worn methods (copied from capitalist and revisionist countries), were trained so-called "first-rate doctors" who were divorced from proletarian politics, divorced from the workers, peasants, and soldiers, and divorced from practice—bourgeois intellectual aristocrats who rode over the working people and thought of nothing else than personal fame, wealth, and position. It ignored the five hundred million peasants and served only the cities. The curriculum required students to study as long as six or even eight years, but after graduation they were unable to treat independently even the most frequently encountered diseases. Leaving the big hospital, with its laboratories and modern equipment, they found themselves at their wits' end. In the course of six years, three fourths of the time was spent studying textbooks and reciting abstract theories. . . .

Even during clinical study and internship they were still taught what had been copied from the capitalist and revisionist countries, such as separating medical science into numerous specialities, with the human body divided into as many airtight compartments. In treatment no consideration was given to what was best for the total patient. Under the domination of bourgeois intellectuals, students concentrated all their energy on the treatment of "rare diseases and difficult cases" and were oblivious of the commonly-seen diseases that most affect the working people. . . .[7]

During the Cultural Revolution, from 1966 to 1969, the medical schools admitted no new classes. Students already in medical school were given accelerated training and then went to work, usually in the countryside.

In the course of the Cultural Revolution higher education of all types underwent major changes in the selection of students and the method and content of the teaching process. Today students generally leave school at age fifteen or sixteen, after completing five years of primary school and three years of junior middle school, and go to work in a commune or factory for two or three years. At the end of that period those who are chosen by their fellow workers, peasants, or soldiers are proposed for admission to universities or professional or technical schools. The criteria by which they are chosen for medical school, for example, are based on political ideology, academic ability, and physical fitness. We were told repeatedly that it is a person's "politics" and his "attitude toward the people" rather than his academic achievement that determines whether he will be a good doctor or other kind of professional. Physical fitness is important, we were told, because being a doctor is such a "strenuous job."

As for the style and content of education, not only was the curriculum generally shortened, but the practical content was markedly increased relative to the theoretical content. Furthermore, periods of direct work are included in all programs. Thus a physics student now spends some time in a factory learning how physics can be applied in production, while a biology student spends time on the communes learning how biology can be helpful in agriculture.

MEDICAL SCHOOLS AFTER THE CULTURAL REVOLUTION

In 1969 the medical schools began to resume admission of new students, but on an experimental basis. In the course of our travels in 1971 we visited and talked with representatives of two medical schools that were functioning again: the Chungshan (Dr. Sun Yat-sen) Medical College in Kwangchow and the Peking Medical College. We also visited two schools, the Shanghai First and Second Medical Colleges, that were still in the process of post-Cultural Revolution reorganization and had not yet admitted new classes. Although we did not visit Tientsin, we talked in Peking with a member of the faculty of the Tientsin Medical College, which was then in the process of admitting its first post-revolution class. During our 1972 trip we talked again with faculty members at Chungshan and at the schools in Peking, where the Peking Second Medical College had resumed classes, and with medical students and faculty in Shanghai. We also visited the Sian Medical College in Shensi Province.

Currently medical education in China is deliberately decentralized and the programs vary widely from city to city, from area to area, and even from school to school within a city. In fact the organization appears to be so decentralized and still so much in flux that we were unable to obtain a complete list of medical schools. A compilation of schools mentioned to us by our various hosts, together with lists published sixteen and nine years ago, respectively, is given in Appendix I.

At the Chungshan Medical College sixty-five students with prior training and experience in health work were admitted in May 1969 to the first experimental class following the Cultural Revolution. They were graduated after one year and sent out to the rural areas where they worked at the production brigade level and in county clinics. They are not, we were told, considered to be fully educated doctors but resemble the "assistant doctors" who, prior to the Cultural Revolution, had received about three years of training. In May 1970 a new class of 600 students was admitted to the school—approximately 350 men and 250 women. These students graduated in 1972 after two years of training. Another class of 600 students was admitted in late 1970, and it is anticipated that they will graduate in three years. On August 15, 1972, another 600 students were admitted.

At the Peking Medical College, after a three-year hiatus 620 students were admitted in December 1970. Of these, 360 are medical students who enrolled in a three-year curriculum (compared to six years before the Cultural Revolution), 120 are pharmacy students in a two-and-a-half year curriculum (compared to five years before), and 140 are nurses undergoing one year of study to qualify as doctors. Two hundred of the 360 medical students are women, and 80 per cent of the students had been barefoot doctors or Red Medical Workers. The college enrolled an additional 432 students on April 17, 1972. At the Tientsin Medical

College, 500 students were admitted in late October 1971; 50 per cent of the entering class were women.

Chang Sin-yen and Li Wei are two examples of medical students at Chungshan. Chang Sin-yen graduated from junior middle school in 1966 at the age of seventeen and went to work in a commune. She was trained as a barefoot doctor and had responsibility for a commune production team of over 100 people. Li Wei graduated from junior medical school in 1967 at age eighteen and was then accepted into the People's Liberation Army where she became a nurse. Both women entered Chungshan Medical College in 1970.

Once a student is chosen by his fellow workers and recommended by the administration of his factory or commune his entrance into medical school must be approved by the administration of the school. We were told that medical schools rarely had any need to exercise a veto because the students' fellow workers "know how to choose those who will make good doctors."

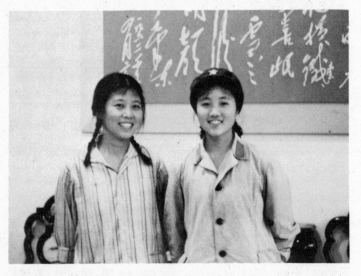

Chang Sin-yen and Li Wei, medical students, Chungshan Medical College.

CURRICULUM AND TEACHING METHODS

Although each medical school has been developing its own independent experimental curriculum since the Cultural Revolution, in 1971 none of the schools we visited expected that the length of "medical training" would extend beyond three years. By the fall of 1972, however, some schools, such as those in Sian and Peking, had instituted a six-month course preceding the formal beginning of the medical curriculum in order to provide additional background in the sciences and in a foreign language.

The 1969 one-year experimental curriculum at Chungshan, for students with previous medical training or experience, was divided into three parts: (1) A combined course in anatomy, histology, biochemistry, and physiology; (2) didactic teaching of clinical subjects; and (3) clinical practice under supervision. The two-year program at Chungshan initiated in May 1970 also began with the same combination course, which lasted three months, followed by a three-month period in which groups of about thirty students went to the countryside with three teachers —two clinicians and a preclinical scientist. The students then returned to the Kwangchow campus where they took a six-month combined course in pharmacology, parasitology, pathology, and physical and laboratory diagnosis. For their second and final year the students took four months in internal medicine and pediatrics, four months in surgery and the surgical specialties, including ten days in ophthalmology, and four months back in the countryside, under supervision, practicing what they had learned. Throughout the two years the students had courses in traditional Chinese medicine and in Mao Tse-tung Thought.

Parenthetically, the introduction of Mao Tse-tung Thought into the medical school curriculum is not a post-Cultural Revolution element. Chi-chao Chan, who studied at Chungshan from 1960 to 1967, and who is now a medical student at Johns Hopkins recalls that:

> Politics always take priority in China. In the first, second, and third years, there were two hours of political lectures per week on the history of the Chinese Communist Party, political economics, and philosophy. In addition, small groups of students met for

political studies two afternoons a week (six hours total) through-out all medical college years. Students criticized each other, read the newspapers, and learned Chairman Mao's works. Each month there was a political meeting for the whole class to summarize the activities that had been carried out since the previous meeting. In addition, every two to three months there was a school-wide meet-ing for the purpose of listening to political reports by the dean or a government officer.[8]

The pattern for an experimental three-year program was presented to us at the Peking Medical College.* The first course, which started in December 1970, lasted about four months and covered anatomy, physiology, biochemistry and histology. This was followed by another four months' course in bacteriology, parasitology, pharmacology, pathology, and laboratory and physi-cal diagnosis. Also covered in the first year was political education and training in aspects of traditional Chinese medicine, including acupuncture. At the end of each year there are two months of physical training, military training, and manual work, and one month's vacation.

In the second and third years the students began their clinical training with courses in internal medicine, pediatrics, surgery, and obstetrics and gynecology in the teaching hospitals; they spend a total of twelve months in the countryside. Because facilities are limited, not all students follow the same schedule, and the periods in the hospitals and in the countryside may be in a different sequence for individual students. All students, however, have the prolonged experience in the countryside work-ing in county and commune hospitals as well as in production brigades. During this period they not only study clinical medicine, but epidemiology, parasitology, environmental sanitation, and other aspects of public health, as well as techniques of traditional Chinese medicine, especially the use of herbs. At the same time, they and their teachers do physical labor in the communes to which they are attached. During the last three months of their third and final year it is planned that students will return to a teaching hospital in Peking where they will consolidate what they

* This curriculum has also been described by E. Grey Dimond.[9]

have learned in the countryside through lectures, discussions, ward rounds, and clinical conferences.

The experimental three-year curriculum at the Tientsin Medical College was described to us by Chu Hsien-yi, its former dean and now a professor in the Department of Endocrinology. The curriculum is similar to that at Peking, with the first year devoted to basic sciences and physical and laboratory diagnoses, and the second to clinical specialties, public health, and traditional medicine. Students spend the first nine months of the third year working in the countryside with their teachers, who supervise the students' practical training and also present theoretical material. The students then return to Tientsin and spend their last three months on the campus and in the teaching hospitals.

When we asked how these schools had managed to compress into three years material that had previously taken six years, we were told, "by eliminating the irrelevant and the redundant, by combining the theoretical with the practical, and by using the 'three-in-one' principle of teachers teach students, students teach teachers, and students teach students." The faculty of the Peking Medical College described in detail the elimination of the irrelevant and the redundant, and told us, for example, in how many different courses they had previously presented material on schistosomiasis. Overall, they said, "we used to require thirty-eight courses to teach a medical student; now we need only ten courses."

We had lengthy discussions about new methods of teaching. We were told that in contrast to the past, students are now encouraged to ask many more questions about what they are being taught, and to participate more actively in the educational process. Students themselves very often take over the teaching role.

In 1971 we were told that there were no grades and no competition. There were indeed examinations in 1971, but solely for the purpose of letting the students know what they had not completely understood, and of letting the teachers know what subjects they were not teaching successfully. We were told there was no reason for grades because classes were small enough, and faculty large enough, for teachers to get to know the students well and be aware of their progress. There is no reason for competition, our hosts stated, because the object is not for individuals to excel but to learn to be good doctors. In 1972, however, we were told that examinations are now given at the end of each course, and that they are graded excellent, good, pass, fail, or on a scale up to 100 points. Our hosts at the Peking Medical College still maintained that there was little competition.

When we asked about dropouts we were told they are extremely rare because "everyone here wants to be a doctor." There is apparently almost no attrition for academic reasons. The only grounds given for students failing to finish medical school is ill health; since 1971 only three students have had to drop out of the Peking Medical College because of illness. When that happens, we were told, the students are encouraged to return to medical school when they recover.

There are no tuition fees, and students are paid a modest stipend (19.50 *yüan* a month in Peking) for living expenses; the amount is sufficient for only a most modest standard of living. There is no charge for books, medical care, or transportation to hospitals or to the countryside. Some entertainment is provided free at the college.

Sian Medical College, established in 1937, grew from a small school with 280 students and a faculty and staff of forty-four before Liberation, to a staff of 2,219 and 2,100 students prior to the Cultural Revolution. The 350 students who comprised the last class prior to the Cultural Revolution were admitted in 1965 and graduated in 1970. In 1972, 568 students were admitted to the first class since the Cultural Revolution. Of this class one-third of the students had completed senior middle school, and two-thirds junior middle school. All have had at least two years of practical experience.

Li Fen, a twenty-two-year-old woman, is one of the new medical students at Sian. She completed senior middle school in 1968 and then went to work in the countryside. When the medical college was about to open, she and nine others from her commune volunteered to attend; four were chosen.

Wang Chen-kang, a twenty-five-year-old student, graduated from junior middle school in 1965. She worked in a county hospital for three years, mostly practicing traditional medicine, prior to joining the People's Liberation Army in 1968 where she continued her medical work. She was interested in attending medical school and was selected by her PLA unit.

After Liu Hsih-yuan graduated from junior middle school in 1963, he engaged in "commercial work" at the county level for two years. He then trained in traditional Chinese medicine from 1965 to 1968 with an old practitioner. Since 1968 Comrade Liu has been providing medical services as a barefoot doctor in a commune. Of the barefoot doctors in his commune, three volunteered to attend medical school; Liu was admitted to Sian Medical College, another to a medical school in Shanghai, and the third to a technical university.

Wang Lai-lin, twenty-five years of age, graduated from junior middle school in 1962 and went on to study traditional and Western medicine in a district hospital. For the past few years he has worked as a barefoot doctor in a commune. More than ten barefoot doctors from his commune volunteered to attend medical school, but only Wang was approved.

As in the other medical schools, in recent years much time has been spent in reevaluating the length and content of the medical curriculum at Sian. Here, too, the six-year program has been reduced to three years. Thirty-one courses have been consolidated into nineteen, and new and more relevant teaching materials have been prepared.

All 568 entering students started with a six-month premedical course consisting of mathematics, physics, chemistry, biology, and a foreign language. The majority of the students are currently studying English, but a few who took Russian in middle school are continuing to do so.

After the premedical course the students began studying anatomy and histology, while continuing with chemistry, physics, and their foreign language. Physiology and biochemistry came somewhat later. In addition, at the beginning of the program students took courses in nursing, primarily supervised by doctors, but sometimes by nurses. During the second term, which began in April or

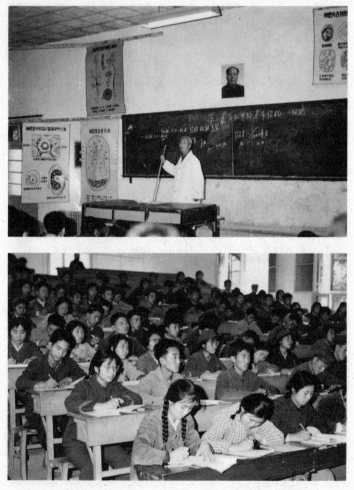

Lecture for first-year students at Sian Medical College.

May 1973, they started to study pathology, pharmacology, and microbiology.

Throughout the first year the students do morning exercises, sports after class, and two hours of gymnastics a week. They also attend classes in Marxism-Leninism-Mao Tse-tung thought. They have a one-month summer vacation in August, and a two-week winter vacation in February.

In October 1973 students at the Sian Medical College will begin a course in the physical examination of patients, to be followed by clinical courses in the various teaching hospitals. In February 1974 teams will go to the countryside for their fourth and fifth terms; the fourth will be spent working together with their teachers, and the fifth in a commune hospital. The students will return to the medical school for the sixth term for further study of ophthalmology, otology, and laryngology. This period will be followed by an internship, after which approximately 10 per cent of the students, those considered suitable to become teachers, will remain for specialized study.

The faculty of the Department of Public Health of the medical college consists of nine members—eight teachers and one technician—who during the third term teach industrial hygiene, statistics, health organization, agricultural and environmental hygiene, nutrition, and care of the newborn. During the fifth term the department conducts courses in medical care organization and "advanced experience."

Members of the department also do research: They visit communes and factories and live with the workers, peasants, and soldiers in order to study and learn their needs more completely. Reports based on this research are subsequently sent to the medical college, the Sian Bureau of Public Health, the local branch of the CMA, and the leaders of the factories and communes. In addition, members of the department study methods of disposal of waste water and residues and prevention of air pollution, and work closely with the city's Bureau of Public Health and medical prevention stations.

A description of the research we observed at the Sian Medical College in 1972 is given in Chapter VIII. Much of the research

in China's medical schools now centers around the techniques of
traditional Chinese medicine, such as acupuncture and the use of
herbs, which are being used in conjunction with Western
medicine.

Since the Cultural Revolution considerable emphasis has
been placed in all medical schools on teaching traditional medicine. In some cities, such as Nanking, the former Chinese (traditional) Medical College has been combined with the Western-type
Nanking Medical College; in others, such as Kwangchow and
Peking, informal arrangements exist between the Western-type and
traditional schools. In these cities some graduates of Western medical colleges may attend traditional colleges for further work after
graduation.

POSTGRADUATE EDUCATION

Postgraduate residency training in clinical specialties still
goes on in China, much as it does in the United States, but with
important differences. Much of the training is provided through
one-year courses in the teaching hospitals. There appear to be far
fewer specialists in training relative to the number of primary
care physicians. Graduates usually do not enter specialty training
until they have spent a period delivering primary care in the
countryside or in a factory. They are chosen for advanced training by the units in which they work, and their salaries are continued during the training period. Reports on a resident's performance during training are sent to his unit and he is expected
to return to the unit upon completion of his residency.

The requirements for completion of specialty training are
set by each hospital on an individual basis, rather than through
national boards. We were told that the length of training is quite
flexible and depends on the abilities of the individual. The physician works much like a "clinical fellow" or a subspecialty resident
in the United States. When his department members—who include nurses, technicians, and others, as well as physicians—make
the decision that he is appropriately trained, he ceases to be a
resident and becomes a full-fledged specialist. In 1972 about 100

postgraduate students were being trained in the four teaching hospitals of the Peking Medical College.

Much stress is now placed on the "reeducation" of urban specialists by means of their being rotated to work in the countryside or in factories. One of the most moving stories of the experience of an urban doctor in the countryside was told us by Chiang Ray-ling, a tall, slim, thirty-seven-year-old female internist at the Friendship Hospital in Peking, who had spent a year with a mobile medical team in Shensi Province. "After the Cultural Revolution started it became clear that conditions in the countryside were more backward than in the cities and that more experienced medical care was needed to serve the peasants," Dr. Chiang told us. Her team was part of the hospital's effort to put resources into rural medical care and to help urban physicians to become more familiar with the peasants' way of life.

Although Dr. Chiang practices only internal medicine in Peking, in the countryside she was called upon to treat all kinds of illnesses; the peasant saw her as a doctor rather than as a specialist. Dr. Chiang lived with the peasants, and ate, worked, and collected medicinal herbs with them. She witnessed "how energetic and how revolutionary their ideology is, and what a heroic spirit they have." Her "sentiments changed" and she started to look upon them as members of her own family. She told us that before her experience in the countryside, when she treated a peasant in the outpatient department she focused only on the disease and not on the patient, or on how he lived or had managed to come to the hospital. Now that she is more familiar with how the peasants live she considers the relationship as being between doctor and patient, not merely between doctor and the patient's disease. Dr. Chiang was in the countryside from May 1970 until July 1971 without once returning to Peking to see her husband and two children, aged eight and two, who were cared for by their grandmother. When we asked why she did not visit her family, she replied, "There was too much work to do."

Finally, continuing education is provided through conferences, and through mutual and self-criticism. Western medical journals and textbooks are available. Publication of Chinese medicaι journals was curtailed during the Cultural Revolution, and, as described elsewhere in this volume, has only recently been resumed. The new *Chinese Medical Journal* stresses technology, to the almost total exclusion of ideology and motivation. It is not yet clear whether all postgraduate education will shift markedly toward the technological, or whether a balance will be found between this and the ideological "service" emphasis of the Cultural Revolution period.

NOTES

1. Chi-Chao Chan, "Medical Education in Mainland China," *Journal of Medical Education* 47 (1972): 327-32.

2. John Z. Bowers, "The Founding of Peking Union Medical College: Policies and Personalities," *Bulletin of the History of Medicine* 45 (1971): 305-21, 409-29.

3. Mary E. Ferguson, *China Medical Board and Peking Union Medical College: A Chronicle of Fruitful Collaboration, 1914-1951* (New York: China Medical Board, 1970).

4. Theodore F. Fox, "The New China: Some Medical Impressions," *The Lancet* 2 (1957): 935-39, 995-99, 1053-57.

5. Revolutionary Committee of China Medical College, Peking, "Thoroughly Criticize and Repudiate the Eight-Year Medical Education Program Pushed by China's Krushchov," *China's Medicine* no. 3 (March 1968): 164-69.

6. Wilder Penfield, "Oriental Renaissance in Education and Medicine," *Science* 141 (1963): 1153-61.

7. Revolutionary Committee of the Shanghai First Medical College, "Medical Education Must be Transformed on the Basis of Mao Tse-tung's Thought," *China's Medicine* 3 (1968): 159-63.

8. Chan, "Medical Education in Mainland China."

9. E. Grey Dimond, "Medical Education and Care in People's Republic of China," *Journal of the American Medical Association* 218 (1967): 1552-57.

VI. Integration of Traditional
and Modern Medicine

THERE are two distinct streams of medicine in China. The Chinese use the term *xiyi* (Western medicine) to differentiate the theory and methods used by doctors trained in "scientific" or "modern" medicine—whether in China or abroad—from those used by doctors trained in *zhongyi* (Chinese medicine).[1,2] Chinese traditional medicine is probably the world's oldest body of medical knowledge, having a history of several thousand years of accumulated empirical observations and abstruse and complex theory.* It incorporates both diagnosis and therapy. Diagnostic methods include observation and questioning of the patient, detailed and prolonged palpation of the pulse, and the use of "diagnostic acupuncture." Therapy makes use of medicinal herbs, moxibustion, breathing and gymnastic exercises, and acupuncture.

The earliest known medical document in what Mao Tse-tung has called the "treasure house of traditional Chinese medicine" is the *Huang-ti Nei-ching* (*The Yellow Emperor's Classic of Internal Medicine*), which popular folklore ascribes to the Yellow Emperor, Huang-ti, who is believed to have lived between 2698 and 2598 B.C. Others maintain that this book, as well as the classic *Shang-han lun* (*Treatise on Fevers*) and *Shen-nung Pen-ts'ao* (*Pharmacopoeia*), was probably written no earlier than the third century B.C., although it may contain theory and practice from much earlier times.

The theoretical concepts of health and disease as expounded in the *Nei-ching* are based for the most part on the notion of

* By virtue of its rich and ancient theoretical base, Chinese traditional medicine differs from many other systems of folk medicine based purely on empirical observations.

127

equilibrium and dynamic balance between opposing forces. For example, *yin* and *yang* are two such principles that permeate all of nature, including biological processes. Health is conceptualized in terms of harmony between the two forces; illness is viewed in terms of an imbalance or disequilibrium. In addition to its theoretical explanation of medical phenomena, the *Nei-ching* includes detailed descriptions of and observations on anatomy, physiology, symptoms of disease, diagnosis, and therapeutic techniques such as moxibustion and acupuncture; the other two classics are less theoretical and contain relatively more empirical information.

The material found in these classics provided the foundation for the traditional medicine that flourished in China for centuries, and that led to a wealth of empirical observations. Among them is said to be the discovery of the circulation of the blood almost 2,000 years before Harvey.[3] The Chinese discovered the fundamentals of smallpox inoculation (variolation) for the prevention of the more serious, naturally acquired smallpox in the middle of the sixteenth century; from China the technique was brought by Russian doctors to Turkey,[4] and from there to England and the West by Lady Mary Wortley Montagu in 1721. It was not until 1798 that Jenner published his observations on cowpox inoculation (vaccination) for the prevention of smallpox.

With the introduction of Western medicine to China, which began in earnest with the missionary efforts of the nineteenth century, there arose great conflicts between the practitioners of the two schools. On the one hand, stories were spread about the "evil practices" of Western doctors; on the other, traditional medicine was condemned as false and superstitious. The Chinese people were often torn between their faith in their traditional medicine and the evidence of the efficacy of Western practices, particularly in surgery and obstetrics. In the cities, while the status and prestige of Western doctors increased relative to those of traditional doctors, there were far too few of them to meet the needs of people, particularly the poor. In the rural areas, except for major provincial towns, Western-type medicine was almost nonexistent.

During the Kuomintang regime, despite the gross shortage of Western-trained doctors, an attempt was made to abolish traditional Chinese medicine. Although this policy failed, the government nonetheless placed many restrictions on the practice of traditional doctors. The Communists were also ambivalent about a practice of medicine that many of the leaders saw as based on superstition, but they did recognize it as the only available source of care for most of China's people.

After Liberation, attempts were made to integrate the work of doctors trained in traditional and Western medicine. In a policy directive to the First National Health Conference in 1950, Mao Tse-tung urged, "Unite all medical workers, young and old, of the traditional and Western schools, and organize a solid united front to strive for the development of the people's health work." [5] And in 1953 he declared, "Chinese medicine and pharmacology are a great treasure house; efforts should be made to explore them and raise them to a higher level." [6]

One of the reasons for urging integration was the belief of many Chinese people that some traditional medical techniques were efficacious and represented a source of medical treatment that should not be discarded. Another reason was that many people, particularly in the rural areas, had so much faith in their traditional doctors that they would sometimes refuse to accept Western practice even when it was available. On more ideological grounds, Croizier attributes the emphasis on Chinese medicine to "cultural nationalism," which has also led to an emphasis on such areas as Chinese painting, music, and drama, as opposed to their Western counterparts. [7] A more pragmatic aspect—and possibly the most important since the Chinese are unashamedly pragmatic in their application of ideology—is the fact that traditional doctors were the only practitioners available in many rural areas. It was therefore considered inevitable that they continue to be used and that they be brought into close contact with Western medicine rather than remain isolated from it.

Whatever the combination of reasons, attempts were made beginning in 1949 to bring the two streams together. The policy was only partly successful, however, and its lack of success was criticized during the Cultural Revolution. Greater efforts at integration have been made in recent years and modern and traditional doctors are now said to have equal rights and status. Each group has been encouraged to learn from the other, and scientific and clinical research is undertaken to achieve a combination of the two approaches that would be superior to either one alone.

During our visits we were able to see a number of examples of the integration of the two types of medicine. Not only are there attempts to combine the techniques, but to coordinate workers in the two disciplines. When we asked about conflicts between the Western-trained and the traditional doctors we were told that both types work together "for the good of the patient"; when disputes arise they can usually be resolved around the needs of the patient.

The question of whether to integrate the body of traditional theory or only the empirically useful remedies of traditional medicine is apparently being actively examined. As in so many other areas, compromises between the extremes are sought. For example, to quote the English summary of an article on "Combined Traditional and Western Medicine in Acute Abdominal Conditions" in the January 1973 issue of the *Chinese Medical Journal:*

> The authors emphasize that, in traditional Chinese medicine, theories (physiology, etiology, pathology), methodology (therapeutic principles), prescriptions, and drugs constitute a unified whole, and methodology is the pivot. The study of methodology will not only reveal the actions of the drugs, but also help to throw light on the nature of the disease itself.
>
> Since medical theory makes constant progress in practice, the authors consider that to examine and employ drugs that show good empirical results, but never neglecting the quest of a scientific explanation of the success, is of tremendous importance in the integration of traditional Chinese medicine and Western medicine.[8]

A number of excellent recent books on traditional Chinese medicine are listed in the bibliography of this volume, and the historical and background material in the remainder of this chapter are drawn from these sources. The material on current practice and current thought in China is drawn from our own experience as well as from recent articles in the *Peking Review, Chinese Medical Journal,* and other Chinese publications.

HERB MEDICINE

Medicines based on ancient herb remedies are widely used in Western medicine. The medicinal uses of the milky sap of unripe seed capsules of the poppy plant were known to the Sumerians in the fourth millenium B.C. The dried sap, known as opium, has been used since the third century B.C. to control diarrhea and alleviate pain, and was part of the armamentarium of Hippocrates. It was not until the nineteenth century that crude opium was purified and its active ingredients, such as morphine, isolated.[9, 10]

Foxglove was mentioned in 1250 in the writings of Welsh physicians, and was described botanically in 1542 under the name *Digitalis purpurea* because the flower resembles a finger and is purple. In 1785 William Withering, an English physician and botanist, described his investigation of a family remedy for dropsy that had long been kept a secret by an old woman in Shropshire. The medicine was composed of twenty or more different herbs, and Withering found that the active herb that was effective as a diuretic was the foxglove. The dried leaf of *Digitalis purpurea,* a flowering biennial indigenous to many areas of the United States, is still used as the official digitalis, although other cardiac glycosides are being used increasingly.[11]

Rauwolfia serpentina is a climbing shrub indigenous to India and its neighboring countries. Its powdered whole root has been used empirically in tropical countries for centuries for a large variety of disorders, especially certain types of insanity. The active alkaloids were not isolated until 1931; reserpine was isolated only in 1952.[12, 13]

The *Shen-nung Pen-ts'ao* contains the names and descriptions of over 350 medications. Among the surviving remedies mentioned is the use of mercury and sulphur for skin diseases. In *Medical Principles and Essentials,* written in about 200 A.D., eighty additional drugs were added, among them, antipyretics, cathartics, diuretics, emetics, sedatives, stimulants, digestive remedies, and antidiarrheal drugs. Centuries later, in 1578, after about thirty years of pharmacological research, Li Shih-chen published his great work, *Compendium of Materia Medica,* in which he listed 1,892 drugs and about 10,000 prescriptions. Among the drugs he enumerated that are still in use are iodine, kaolin, ephedrine, *Dichoroa febrifuga* for malaria, and *Mylitta lapidescens* for tapeworm.[14, 15]

The ancient Chinese, as did other peoples, seized upon many herbs for superstitious reasons. For example, a plant was supposed to be effective against diseases of an organ whose shape it resembled, or if the name of the disease resembled that of the plant. The popular Chinese ginsing root is a case in point: The root, like the European mandrake, resembles the shape of a man— the two tips of the root look like legs and the two upper continuums resemble arms. Although there is no evidence that the plant, celebrated as the "herb of eternal life," indeed gives immortality, it is reported to increase sexual powers, "tonify" the central nervous system, and "regulate" the blood pressure. The herb is widely used in China and elsewhere, but an active principle has yet to be isolated.

On the other hand, the herb *ma huang* (ephedra) is an example of a Chinese medicinal herb that has yielded an active isolate widely accepted in modern medicine. Translated as "yellow astringent," *ma huang* has been used by traditional physicians in the treatment of pulmonary and other diseases for thousands of years. Reference to it is found in the *Shen-nung Pen-ts'ao* and the *Compendium of Materia Medica,* where it is described as valuable as an antipyretic, diaphoretic, circulatory stimulant, and sedative for cough.

The active principle of *ma huang* was first isolated in 1885. In 1887 the active alkaloid, ephedrine, was obtained in pure form and introduced to medical science by the Japanese as a mydriatic (pupil dilater) in the treatment of eye diseases. It fell into disuse shortly thereafter, and it was not until 1925 that modern medicine rediscovered its use in the treatment of asthma. Throughout this time, however, traditional Chinese medical practitioners had continued to use the herb.[16]

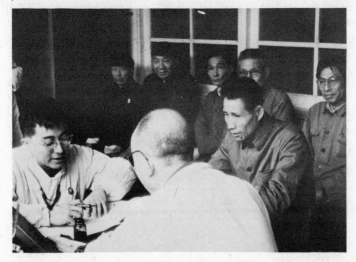

A doctor of Western medicine (left) and of traditional Chinese medicine (back to camera) with patients in the hypertension clinic, Juichin Hospital, Shanghai.

The traditional Chinese classification of medications is divided into three main groups; those of vegetable, animal, and mineral origin. The first of these is the most important. An example of the second is the use of the dried skin of the common toad, *ch'an su*, for toothache and bleeding gums. It was only recently demonstrated that toad skin contains a high percentage of epinephrine, a hemostatic when used locally.

The use of herb medicine, as with other therapeutic methods, was in part found in the complex theories of traditional Chinese medicine. But even more important, apparently, was the empirical knowledge of medicinal herbs gained by popular experience.

In contemporary China traditional herb medicines are used universally—we saw numerous examples of this in the smallest production brigade health station in the communes and the largest hospital in Shanghai. In the communes the barefoot doctors and other peasants gather, and at times themselves grow, herbs for medicinal use that are then prepared and stored. Red Medical

Workers are urged to grow, collect, and use herbs. Most herb medicines are given in the form of tea or a broth made by boiling the herb in water. In some communes we observed apparatuses used for extraction of active principles from the herbs.

The herb medicines are used, in combination with Western-style medicines, by barefoot doctors, traditional doctors, and Western doctors. In Shanghai's Juichin Hospital, we observed a traditional doctor and Western doctor together examining a patient with hypertension and together prescribing a combination of modern and traditional medicines to lower the blood pressure.

Specific examples of herbs currently being used are given in the first issue of the recently resumed *Chinese Medical Journal.* For example, six traditional prescriptions are described as "effective in the treatment of acute abdominal conditions," [17] and "more than twenty specific drugs that can 'tonify the heart and disperse the disease factors' " [18] were used in patients with acute myocardial infarction.

Research workers in the Institute of Materia Medica in Peking are attempting to isolate and identify the active principles in herb medicines. The institute, which is under the aegis of the Chinese Academy of Medical Sciences, has departments of pharmaceutical chemical synthesis, phytochemistry, pharmacological analysis, and pharmacological research.

Among the substances being studied is *Securinega suffruticos* from which an alkaloid, securinine, is extracted and purified. This alkaloid is being subjected to clinical trial in the treatment of chronic paralysis following Bell's palsy, and paralysis following poliomyelitis. Another herb being used is *Thevetja peruviana,* a crude plant that grows widely in China, whose dried seeds are being used for the extraction of nerifolin, a rapid-acting digitalis glycoside, which is now being produced commercially in China, thus eliminating the need to import strophanthin. [19]

Despite the efforts of this and other institutes, most of the herb medicines currently used in China remain unrefined and, in the Western "scientific" sense, unevaluated. Our hosts believe that these medicines will continue to be used because of the Chinese people's and most practitioners' faith in them and the empirical evidence of their efficacy, and that it will be many years—if ever—before they will be subjected to "double-blind," randomized, controlled clinical trials of the type that are increasingly an article of faith in the West.

TREATMENT OF FRACTURES

The first Chinese medical treatise on the treatment of fractures appeared in the ninth century A.D., and the principles laid down in it are still used in China. The management of certain fractures differs from that in the United States, where not only the fracture itself, but the joints adjoining it are usually immobilized in a plaster cast. In the traditional Chinese method, the fracture is maintained in alignment, often by a splint, while the neighboring joints are left free for early exercise. In the United States the reduction of a fracture by bringing the two ends of the broken bone into realignment is often done in a single forcible movement, sometimes under anesthesia. The Chinese method obtains the realignment gradually, without the use of anesthesia.

Joshua Horn, the British orthopedist who spent fifteen years practicing in China, points out that there are advantages and disadvantages to both methods and that active attempts are being made to combine the advantages of both. Some drawbacks he found with the traditional method were: it is not always possible to reduce a fracture without anesthesia; it is sometimes difficult to prevent redisplacement after reduction; oblique and fragmented fractures sometimes unite with excessive shortening; if the splints are tied too tightly a sloughing of the soft tissue may result; and the process is time consuming.[20] Some of the benefits Chinese physicians find in the traditional method are: it provides a satisfactory reduction of the fracture; a more rapid recovery of function is obtained; and the treatment has a shorter course than with modern methods. Nonunion or delayed union of the bone rarely occurs.[21]

Combining the advantages of both traditional and modern treatments depends to a large extent on the nature of the particular fracture. In some cases, aspects of both methods are combined throughout; others are treated first by the modern and then

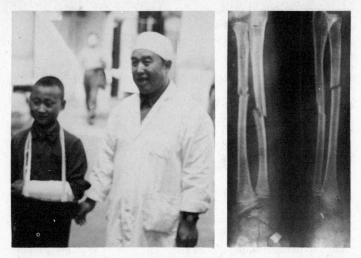

Thirteen-year old boy, with fracture of both bones of his left forearm, with limb in traditional Chinese splint; on his left is the head of the Traditional Bone Department, Fengsheng neighborhood hospital, Peking. X-ray on right shows good apposition of the fracture fragments.

by the traditional method; still others are treated solely by one method. An example of traditional treatment was shown us in the Traditional Bone Department of the Fengsheng neighborhood hospital in Peking. The patient was a thirteen-year-old boy who had fractured both bones of his left forearm while playing basketball, and who was being treated by a traditional Chinese physician. The X-ray of the fractures shows that the bones are being retained in good apposition by the splinting.

Horn gives an example of combining the two methods in his discussion of the treatment of fractures that have a tendency to shorten. These fractures are treated by a period of traction, as in the United States, but combined with traditional splintage and early exercise of the injured limb. This integration of methods results, Horn states, in a considerably shorter duration of traction and a more rapid healing than would occur with modern methods alone.[22]

An example of the use of the traditional method only is seen in the treatment of a Colles' fracture of the wrist. In order to achieve immobilization, Chinese doctors use pliable willow-wood splints, each of which is lined with a thin layer of felt. After the fracture has been reduced, the splints are taped over the wrist; this fixation permits the wrist to move freely in the palmer and ulnar directions, and leaves all fingers free to move. There is thus an early institution of active motion of the wrist and the fingers. The motion is said to promote reduction of swelling, prevent adhesion and pressure sores, and help to reduce any further displacement that may be present after the reduction. In a series of 100 cases reported in the *Chinese Medical Journal* in 1964, the authors indicated that the results were better than in other series using Western methods.[23] In the Friendship Hospital in Peking we were introduced to a Western-type neurologist wearing a willow-wood splint for her Colles' fracture.

Moxibustion

The theory of the interconnection between internal organs and sites on the skin is to be found in the *Nei-ching,* along with theories of channels or meridians (*chinglo*) running throughout the body, close to the skin.[24] Stimulation of these sites by inserting needles (acupuncture) or by applying heat (moxibustion) is said to produce therapeutic effects. A few of the connections have been "confirmed," both theoretically and empirically, by Western neurologists. For example, in 1898 Henry Head, an English neurologist, reported a connection between zones on the skin, which are named after him, and certain organs. When the organs are diseased, pain is referred to the zones on the skin.[25] For the most part, however, there are no known neurological pathways between the points on the skin and the internal organs with which they are traditionally associated.

In traditional moxibustion therapy the leaves of the mugwort plant, *Artemisia vulgaris,* or moxa, are dried for three years, pulverized into a fine powder, and then wrapped in paper in the shape of a cone, a ball, or a stick. The moxa is set either directly or indirectly on points of the skin, ignited, and, in former times, left to burn down to the skin.[26] In the indirect method, which is said to be more common now, a herbal insulator such as ginger or garlic is placed between the moxa and the skin. In our few observations of moxibustion the aim seemed to be to produce warmth rather than burning. In one demonstration we witnessed, on the sprained ankle of a Western visitor, the burning moxa was simply held near the hemarthrosis, providing what a Western orthopedist might call "local dry heat."

MASSAGE

Traditional Chinese medicine has for thousands of years used massage not only to relieve local pain but for therapeutic treatment of diseases of internal organs. In the latter case, stimulation is applied to the same points on the body surface as are used in moxibustion and acupuncture. Several different forms of massage are used for adults; others are recommended for children.[27]

Through the centuries the use of massage has been accompanied by many mystical elements. Contemporary medical researchers, however, are apparently removing these elements and combining massage with other therapeutic techniques. For example, in the Shanghai Sanatorium for Respiratory Therapy, massage as a supplementary therapeutic technique was found to be beneficial.[28]

EXERCISE

As early as the third century B.C., inscriptions found on jade stones revealed that the ancient Chinese recommended breathing exercises to promote longevity. Under the influence of Taoism, breathing exercises were first used as a form of therapy for various diseases. The *Nei-ching* describes the therapeutic potential of respiratory exercises. With the introduction of Buddhism in the first century A.D., breathing exercises were used for the achievement of a spiritual state, as in Indian yoga, rather than for specifically medical purposes. These exercises require the full concentration of the individual. Some of the special features of traditional breathing exercises involve the active participation of

the patient in helping to cure his own illness; the close relationship between the patient and the therapist who teaches the
exercises; the patient's mental state—the desired resultant psychic
state is one of repose and equilibrium; and the requirement of
periods of rest.[29] An important current use of breathing exercises
is in the preparation of patients for open-chest surgery,[30] which is
described in the section on acupuncture anesthesia (see page 147).

Chinese gymnastic exercises are simple and do not demand
extreme exertion or bodily contortions. Their aim is to relax
physiological and psychological tensions. The exact movements are
prescribed in detail and must be followed methodically. As with
breathing exercises they can be performed accurately only under
the guidance of an instructor. Again the individual's mental
state is an important component and care is taken that he is not
distracted. Gymnastic exercises are used as an adjunct treatment
for high blood pressure, tubercular infection, digestive disorders,
and paralysis.[31]

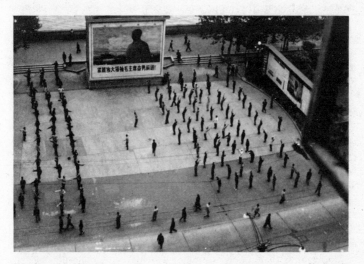

Workers in Shanghai square at 7:30 A.M. doing Western calisthenics
(right) and traditional Chinese exercises (left).

The Chinese, as do we, consider gymnastic exercises as an important component in preventive medicine—to maintain and enhance physical fitness. We observed people all over China— including office workers in Shanghai at 7:30 A.M., before they started their day's work—performing both traditional Chinese exercises and Western-style calisthenics.

ACUPUNCTURE IN DIAGNOSIS AND TREATMENT

In traditional Chinese medicine, acupuncture—the insertion of fine metal needles into strategic groups of points on the body, often distant from the target organ—has been used to treat a wide variety of illnesses. The acupuncture points on the skin are, according to the theory, the spots where the meridians (*chinglo*) emerge on the surface. The theory states that the ebb and flow of the vital forces occurs along these meridians and are intricately interconnected with the internal organs and points on the skin. The insertion of needles into these sites is said to equalize the balance between the opposing forces and cause therapeutic changes in the affected organ. The place and depth of insertion, type of needle used (there are nine classic shapes), and the duration of insertion are determined in relation to the affected organ.[32]

The number of sites at which acupuncture treatment is said to be effective is increasing from the classic 295 (or 365, 649, 657, or 667, depending on the source one uses) points. In 1971 Palos stated that "today some 722 points are generally acknowledged." [33] Whereas ancient Chinese medicine considered a wide range of spots on the skin to be forbidden, contemporary writers have different opinions. New methods of acupuncture added in recent years not only include

> . . . new points of insertion and, on occasion, deeper placement, but also constant manipulation of the needle. This manipulation of the needle can be described as a rapid up-and-down traverse of the needle over a distance of approximately one-half inch, simultaneous with a rapid to-and-fro twirling of the needle by the thumb and fingers. The up-and-down motion is at approximately 120 "cycles" per minute.[34]

The effects of acupuncture therapy are most difficult to explain when they occur far from the point of the needle's insertion. For example, migraine headache is treated by inserting needles at points in the hands or feet; and some forms of heart disease, at points on the back of the arms.

Needling the *hoku* point, between the metacarpi of the thumb and forefinger, is said to be especially effective for toothaches, and needling the *tsusanli* point, on the external side of the leg just below the knee, is good for gastrointestinal diseases.[35]

In addition, under fluoroscopic examination it has been found that stimulation of the *tsusanli* point of either a human or animal subject intensifies intestinal peristalsis.

Dramatic effects in the treatment of deafmutes by acupuncture have recently been reported. The use of acupuncture in such treatments is said to have been discovered as recently as 1968 by army medical teams in northeast China. "Deep needling of the *yamen* point, for instance, enables deaf-mutes to hear and speak." [36] As is the case with other innovative procedures in acupuncture, the medical workers used their own bodies for experimentation; after repeated self-experimentation, they are said to have located the points that appear to affect hearing.[37]

Currently, acupuncture is widely used in China in the treatment of a great variety of conditions. We personally observed dysmenorrhea being treated by the insertion of needles into the lower legs. Another new method is to combine acupuncture with electrical stimulation from DC pulsators using batteries (see Appendix J). Such therapy was being given in the treatment of peripheral vascular disease (hardening of the arteries of the legs) at the Juichin Hospital in Shanghai. We were told that in a series of cases in which the disease was treated by this method there was some subjective relief of symptoms in 84 per cent of the patients, and objective changes in pulses in 30 per cent.

At the Bethune International Peace Hospital in Shihkiachwang, a number of diseases and impairments are being treated experimentally with acupuncture. We saw treatments being given to patients with psoriasis and other skin diseases, headaches, and paralysis secondary to stroke. Other conditions for which acu-

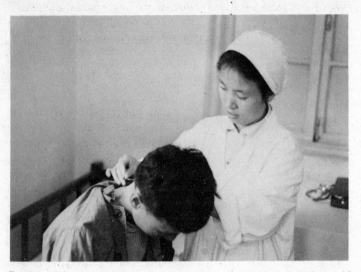

Doctor giving acupuncture treatment at the Peking Printing and Dyeing Mill.

puncture is used at the hospital, we were told, include paralysis secondary to poliomyelitis or spinal cord tumor, peripheral neuritis, sciatica, retinitis, epilepsy, Meniere's syndrome, and hysteria.

Among the reasons acupuncture is used so widely is its inexpensiveness and its safety. We were told repeatedly how few complications or dangerous side effects result from acupuncture treatments. It should not be assumed, however, that acupuncture treatment is completely benign. An article in the December 1964 issue of the *Kiangsu Journal of Chinese Traditional Medicine* describes eight cases of accidental damage to internal organs due to acupuncture.[38] In two cases the damage led to deaths, in the other six it was necessary to repair a peritoneal tear, perform arterial ligation, thoracic surgery, and gallbladder surgery, remove a spleen, and remove a kidney.

In 1965 an article in the *Kwangtung Medical Journal*—

Chinese Traditional Medicine described four cases of serious bacterial infection following the use of acupuncture.[39] Although all the infections were reversed by the use of antibiotics, the author warns against the use of unsterilized needles on undisinfected skin, and urges the application of a "hemostat" after acupuncture treatment. Other possible dangers include the spread of hepatitis through the use of unsterilized needles, and a concern that many American physicians have expressed about its uncritical use: the masking of symptoms of an underlying disorder at a time when it might still be potentially reversible or curable.

We did not observe some of the other uses of acupuncture about which the Chinese have been writing recently. In some cases of poliomyelitis or paraplegia it has been reported that a series of acupuncture treatments can restore the function of limbs paralyzed for years.[40] In 1971 the *Peking Review* presented a brief article entitled, "Treating Acute Abdominal Cases without Operations:" [41]

> Combining traditional Chinese and Western medicine, China's medical workers have had initial good results in treating acute abdominal cases without operating.
> The cases include acute appendicitis, intestinal obstruction, pancreatitis, perforation of the ulcer [sic], cholecystitis (inflammation of the gall bladder), gallstone, biliary ascariasis (parasitic roundworm in the bile duct), ectopic pregnancy, etc. In place of operations, traditional Chinese and Western medicine for both internal and external purposes, injections and acupuncture are used in most cases. A number of successes have been reported in many places.
> In April this year, Yao Ching-lu, an old peasant on Tientsin's outskirts, had an acute appendicitis with complications of diffuse peritonitis. When he was rushed to the hospital, intestinal paralysis occurred and the case was critical. The doctors treated him by acupuncture and gave him Chinese medicine both internally and externally in coordination with infusions and other methods. The pain eased the same day. The following day abdomen tension was less. He began eating the fourth day and was discharged fully recovered on the tenth day. . . .
> Statistics in Tientsin's Nankai Hospital show that since 1962, 80 per cent of the patients with acute appendicitis have been cured without an operation. The percentage is over 90 for patients with

acute pancreatitis and biliary ascariasis and 70 and over 50 in
acute perforations of ulcers and acute intestinal obstruction, respectively. In the hospital attached to the Tsunyi Medical College,
success was reported in some 90 per cent of the 1,500 acute abdominal cases treated without being operated on in the last two
years. In the past decade or so one hospital in Shansi Province has
saved the lives of 520 women with cases of ectopic pregnancy without an operation and their ability to give birth not affected.

It is not clear to what extent these reported successes depend
on acupuncture, herb medicines, and Western-type antibiotics and
other medications, or on the combination of the three. What is
clear is that acupuncture as a method of treating painful conditions has had a long and apparently successful history and holds
an honored place in medical care in the People's Republic of
China. But evaluation of the results achieved by acupuncture treatment is apparently still inadequate, at least according to Western
ideas of how such data should be recorded and evaluated.

ACUPUNCTURE ANESTHESIA

Acupuncture anesthesia—the use of acupuncture to induce
analgesia during surgery—is a technique that was introduced in
China in about 1958. While it is still in the experimental stage
and used in only a small fraction of operations performed in
China, it is viewed by the Chinese as an excellent example of
success in the integration of traditional and modern medicine.

In 1971 it was reported that "over 400,000 patients have
received acupuncture anesthesia for more than a hundred different
major and minor operations. The ratio of effectiveness is around
90 per cent." [42] We were told in Peking, however, that this
percentage does not always represent "total success," and that in
some cases pain is felt. Considerable research on acupuncture
anesthesia is currently underway, some of it by medical workers
experimenting on themselves, to determine the reasons for its
success and to improve the technique.

A few years ago, analgesia was induced by needling only those
points on the patient's body described in traditional Chinese
medical literature; it has now been extended to other areas—the
ears, nose, and other parts of the face. Electric stimulation through

the needles has been added to the repertoire of the acupuncture anesthetist. Also added has been the use of local anesthetic drugs and/or massage at supplementary acupuncture sites.

The number of essential points of insertion to induce anesthesia has been reduced. Formerly a patient undergoing a pneumonectomy had to be needled at several dozen, and sometimes more than 100, points, which required four acupuncturists constantly manipulating needles. After first experimenting on themselves, medical workers have been able to reduce the number of points "to a few and sometimes even to one." [43] Since the degree of analgesia appears to be similar, even with the reduction of sites, this, as well as the electrical stimulation that is replacing manual manipulation, has been a great advance in the technique.

We had an opportunity to observe several operations using acupuncture anesthesia at the Third Teaching Hospital attached to the Peking Medical College, where the acupuncture anesthesia group is a subdivision of the anesthesiology department. Between 1958 and July 1971 acupuncture anesthesia had been used on 4,900 cases at this hospital. The operations included ophthalmological, thyroidectomy, ENT, open-chest, gastrectomy, cholecystectomy, appendectomy, and operations on the limbs. In each case, we were told, it was necessary to have the full cooperation of the patient—if he was too anxious, a general anesthetic was used.

We watched the surgery from over the shoulders of the surgeons, from overhead observations balconies, or over closed-circuit television. Among the operations we observed were: The removal of a tumor from the left frontal cerebral lobe of a forty-year-old woman; the removal of the tuberculous left upper lobe of the lung of a man of thirty-two; and the removal of an ovarian cyst from a woman aged thirty-one. These operations have also been described in detail by Dimond.[44]

The preoperative drugs used for the woman undergoing removal of the tumor were phenobarbital sodium and atropine the night before surgery, and mannitol to decrease intracranial pressure. Three stainless steel acupuncture needles were inserted in different places on the head, and a metal plate was attached

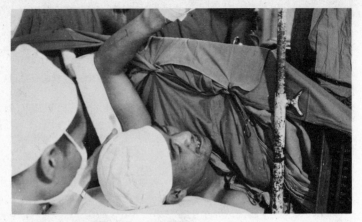

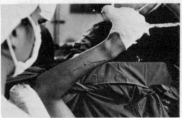

Patient undergoing pulmonary lobectomy under acupuncture anesthesia produced by a single needle in his left forearm. Close-up of the needle in place is at bottom.

to the back of the head (the occiput). A pulse generator was attached to the needles, delivering 9 v. at from 120 to 180 cycles/minute. The patient was conscious but barely able to speak or respond to stimuli; no evidence of pain was observed.

The anesthesia for the patient undergoing the pulmonary lobectomy required only one needle, about one-and-one-half inches long, inserted about 2 cm. into his left forearm between the wrist and elbow. An injection of 10 mg. of morphine sulphate was given about half an hour before the incision in an acupuncture site on the left side of his neck. After twenty minutes of manipulating the needle the two-hour operation began; throughout there was much conversation between the patient, himself a surgeon, and the surgeons performing the operation. The patient showed no evidence of pain and in the middle of the operation there was a break while he ate some fruit.

We have frequently been asked since our return how it was possible for open-chest surgery to be performed without tracheal intubation and positive pressure respiration.* An explanation was given in a recent issue of *Peking Review*,[45] quoted here in full:

> The development of chest surgery is closely related to improvement in the instruments and technique for giving the patient positive pressure breathing. Before the surgeons mastered this technique, it was very dangerous to perform chest surgery under normal atmospheric pressure.
>
> When we first began performing a pneumonectomy under acupunctural anesthesia, apart from inserting needles in those points which induce analgesia, we also inserted needles in the points which could improve the patient's breathing in order to avoid physiological breathing disorders due to the sudden opening of the chest. With this method, although no danger emerged due to atelectasis, the patient still had difficulty in breathing.
>
> To solve this problem we injected air into the side of the chest to be operated on to deflate the lung beforehand in order to create artificial atelectasis. This enabled the patient to adapt to comparatively strong air pressure when the chest was opened during the operation. This still could not solve mediastinal flutter— big vibration of some organs in the chest cavity following a shortage of breath—and disorder in breathing.
>
> In addition to acupunctural anaesthesia, we applied the breathing therapy of traditional Chinese medicinal practice. Before the operation, we asked the patient to practice deep abdominal breathing. Because breathing was mainly compensated for by the other lung, slow abdominal breathing by the patient during the operation and full function of the other lung helped maintain his breathing and overcome flutters of the organs so as to facilitate the operation.
>
> Performing a pneumonectomy under acupunctural anaesthesia is being continually developed and perfected. A patient previously had to be needled at forty points on his limbs, and four medical workers had to twirl the needles without let-up during the operation. The number of points needled gradually has been re-

* The opening of the chest to atmospheric pressure not only collapses the lung on the side of the chest that is open but permits shifting and instability of the midline structures (mediastinum), which often causes problems in breathing with the other lung.

duced to sixteen, then twelve and, later, only two. In the past year
or so, we have successfully performed more than 100 lung operations by deeply inserting only one needle on the external side of
the patient's forearm involving two points.

There are still some problems to be handled in thoracic
operations under acupunctural anesthesia. The question we are
now studying is how to perform an operation on a patient with a
low pulmonary function.

The patient we observed undergoing removal of an ovarian
cyst received phenobarbital sodium; just before surgery a small
dose of scopolamine was injected at an acupuncture point on each
leg. Needles placed on either side of the lumbar spine area and
on each leg were attached to two 9-v. electrostimulators, one for
the needles in the back and one for those in the legs. This was
the only surgery we witnessed in which the anesthesia was not
fully satisfactory. The woman obviously felt considerable pain
when the cyst was being removed, and at this point the surgeons
administered "novocaine" (procaine hydrochloride) into the
peritoneal cavity, and an acupuncture needle was inserted in her
ear.* The operation then proceeded without further anesthesia
and the patient showed little evidence of pain. The surgeons
explained to us that acupuncture anesthesia was "much more
successful in surgery above the waist than in surgery below the
waist."

At a postsurgical conference at the Peking Third Hospital we
were told that the point at which the anesthesiologist knows he is
in the right place is when the patient has a feeling of "distention."
The surgeon is also said to feel something when he arrives at the
right place, but this was hard to define: it was variously called
"resistance," "heaviness," and "stickiness."

We asked about the importance of reassurance, talking to the
patient, and about the attention given to the patient. They
responded that an operation is a big event and that the patient
must have worries about it and is probably afraid of pain. If the
patient is "too anxious," acupuncture anesthesia is not used even

* Acupuncture is also used for other complications in abdominal surgery; for
example, needling at the *chuehmen* point is used to control spasm of the diaphragm
if it occurs during splenectomy.[46]

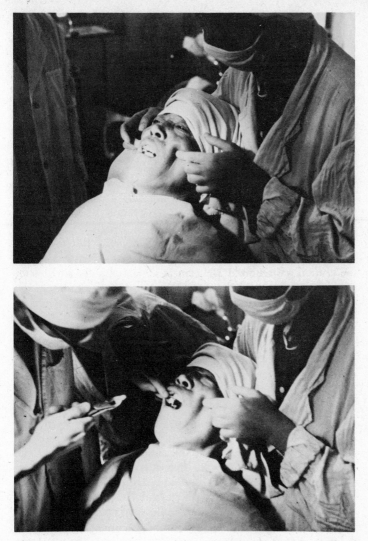

Patient having tooth extracted under acupuncture anesthesia produced by finger pressure.

if the patient asks for it. During acupuncture anesthesia it is very important to reassure the patient and to tell him that he and the doctor will fight together against pain and disease. There is usually almost constant conversation between the patient and the acupuncturist.

In a dental clinic in Shanghai we observed anesthesia produced by finger pressure at acupuncture points, without the use of needles. Pressure was applied for about one minute, a tooth was extracted, and the patient insisted—under our incredulous cross-examination—that he had felt no pain.

Acupuncture anesthesia is practiced in several of China's hospitals, including many outside the large cities. For example, we observed a partial gastrectomy for ulcers conducted under acupuncture anesthesia at the Bethune Hospital. The patient, a thirty-three-year-old man, had six needles inserted—two in the legs, two in the neck, and two in the abdomen—with each pair attached to DC stimulators. We were told that no other analgesic medication was required. Dr. Han Hsin-mian, the female director of the anesthesia department, told us that the two needles in the neck would have been removed had the patient felt completely comfortable, but since he felt some discomfort they were retained.

Physicians in China listed for us many advantages of acupuncture anesthesia: It is simple, safe, economical, and usually effective; recovery from surgery and wound-healing are said to be faster; the patient can eat immediately following or even during most surgery, and there is no vomiting afterwards; there is less secondary infection; and since the patient is conscious he can act in coordination with the doctor in the regulation of normal functions. In certain operations, such as removal of an acoustic neuroma, it is very helpful if the patient is conscious and can describe certain sensations so that the surgeon can avoid inadvertently damaging other cerebral nerve tissue.[47] The harmful side effects of general anesthesia are avoided, which is especially important if a patient is sensitive to the drugs being used.

The only two unsatisfactory aspects of acupuncture anesthesia mentioned to us are the later soreness for up to one or two days at the points where the needles were inserted, and the occasional failure of the technique in particular patients or in certain kinds of surgery, so that general anesthesia or other analgesics must be used.

Research on methods of action of acupuncture anesthesia was described by the Peking Acupunctural Anesthesia Coordinating Group in a recent article in *Peking Review*.[48] Acupuncture is said to have two major physiological effects: (1) "Analgesic effect": the pain threshold has been measured in both man and animals and found to be elevated by acupuncture; recent experimentation has indicated that the electroencephalographic changes caused by painful stimuli in animals could be weakened or entirely suppressed by acupuncture; and (2) "regulating effect": the article states that acupuncture

> . . . restores the disrupted functions of the human body to normal. Clinically, we often find that needling the same point corrects both diarrhea and constipation, and brings a rapid or slow heart rate back to normal. Needling is good for high or low blood pressure, helps those who have fainted or are in a state of shock to regain consciousness, provides sedation for the agitated and helps those suffering from insomnia to get a good sleep. Needling is also efficacious for certain cases of inflammation. Experimental study has shown that needling certain points on the body of a normal person or animal increases the number of white blood corpuscles and intensifies phagocytosis.

The Peking anesthesiologists believe that these two effects reinforce each other. Another element is the patient's "initiative." Although "the patient's initiative alone cannot replace acupunctural anesthesia . . . acting together the two can raise the patient's threshold for pain." The anesthesiologists urged that ". . . while we gradually improve acupunctural anesthesia through practice we should carry out careful and painstaking scientific research."

One of the research questions currently being studied in China is: What is the nature of the specific association, if any, between the skin sites and the internal organs affected? Modern neurophysiological theory insists on finding anatomically demonstrable nerve pathways. Chinese research workers are asking to what extent the traditional *chinglo* meridians and nerve pathways are actually the same. After making "a correlative analysis

of the results of acupuncture anesthesia and segmental inner-
vation," they found that while the two in large measure correspond
to one another, they are not identical. They concluded that
chinglo probably includes not only the nerve pathways, but
"blood vessels and endocrine structures and some of their functions." The *chinglo* relationships cannot be entirely accounted
for by current knowledge of neuroanatomy and neurophysiology.
For example, based on the *chinglo* theory, empirical needling of
the *kuangming* point in the leg has produced analgesia for eye
operations, even though there are no known nerve pathways
between the *kuangming* point and the eye. It is of interest,
though the relevance is not clear, that Russian researchers on
Kirlian photography, a technique using a high frequency electrical field, have recently found peculiar flaring effects on the
skin that are concentrated on those areas of the body that traditional Chinese medicine has identified as acupuncture points; [49]
thus the acupuncture points may indeed have some special
anatomical characteristics not yet determined.

Current research at the Shanghai Institute of Physiology,
according to reports of visitors in early 1973, is pursuing another
line, one that requires no specific connection between the skin
site and the target organ. The investigators hypothesize that acupuncture acts on the proprioceptors—muscles spindles and related
stretch and pressure receptors. The nerve impulses over this path-
way then act, by a kind of relatively nonspecific competitive
inhibition at the spinal cord or thalamic level, to block the
sensation carried over the pain pathways.[50] This idea of competitive
inhibition blocking pain sensation is in some ways related to a
theory known as the "gate-control theory of pain," put forth in
the West by Melzack, Wall,[51, 52] and other workers. The Shanghai
investigators emphasize that their explanation of the phenomenon
is at best partial and incomplete, and that many aspects of the
effect of acupuncture remain to be explained.

Many Western physicians remain skeptical and consider acupuncture to be a "placebo" or a form of "hypnosis"; some even
maintain it does not work at all and that those who report that
it does have been "duped." [53,54] Insofar as this skepticism is based

on the absence of a full "causal" or "scientific" explanation, as opposed to the absence of controlled clinical trials, it seems to us unjustified. The absence of a causal explanation does not mean that a technique does not work or that there are no direct physiological or pharmacological effects. We in the "scientific" West use aspirin to good effect even though there are conflicting and as yet unproven theories about "how" it works; [55] few would ascribe its effects to placebo or hypnotic mechanisms.

We are convinced that acupuncture does "work" in China. The evidence that it produces analgesia during surgery is clear to the observer; the evidence that it works in the treatment of medical problems, particularly painful ones, is less clear in the absence of controlled trials. But the testimony of patients about immediate effects, and the survival of the technique over two millenia suggest considerable efficacy. Although there is no doubt in our minds that acupuncture, both as a treatment and in surgical anesthesia, works in China, the extent to which the technique is transplantable to the United States is a much more complex question. It is well known that much medical treatment, including a significant portion of the effects of powerful drugs such as morphine, depends for its effectiveness on the faith of the healer and/or the patient that it will work. Without denigrating the physiological effects of acupuncture, which we believe exist even though a full "scientific" explanation has not yet been found, it still remains to be seen how effective it will be—and under what circumstances—in a society lacking over twenty centuries of faith in it.

NOTES

1. Ralph C. Croizier, *Traditional Medicine in Modern China* (Cambridge: Harvard University Press, 1968).

2. ———, "Traditional Medicine as a Basis for Chinese Medical Practice," in *Medicine and Public Health in the People's Republic of China*, ed. Joseph R. Quinn (Washington, D.C.: Department of Health, Education, and Welfare Publication #NIH 72-67, 1972).

3. ———, *Traditional Medicine in Modern China*, p. 121.

4. Stephan Palos, *The Chinese Art of Healing* (New York: Herder and Herder, 1971): p. 15.

5. Joshua S. Horn, *Away with All Pests . . . An English Surgeon in People's China* (New York: Monthly Review Press, 1969): p. 76.

6. "China Creates Acupunctural Anesthesia," *Peking Review* 14, no. 33 (1971): 7-9.

7. Croizier, *Traditional Medicine in Modern China*, p. 4.

8. "Combined Traditional and Western Medicine in Acute Abdominal Conditions," (abstracts) *Chinese Medical Journal* no. 1 (1973): 8.

9. Louis S. Goodman and Alfred Gilman, *The Pharmacological Basis of Therapeutics*, 2nd. ed. (New York: Macmillan, 1955): p. 216.

10. Joseph R. DiPalma, ed., *Drill's Pharmacology in Medicine* (New York: McGraw-Hill, 1965): p. 248.

11. Goodman and Gilman, *The Pharmacological Basis*, p. 668-69.

12. Ibid., p. 754.

13. DiPalma, *Drill's Pharmacology*, p. 349.

14. Horn, *Away with All Pests*, pp. 74-75.

15. Chang Hui-chien, *Li Shih-chen—Great Pharmacologist of Ancient China* (Peking: Foreign Languages Press, 1960).

16. Goodman and Gilman, *The Pharmacological Basis*, p. 505-506.

17. "Combined Traditional and Western Medicine."

18. "Acute Myocardial Infarction Treated with Traditional and Western Medicine," *Chinese Medical Journal* no. 1 (January, 1973): 7.

19. E. Grey Dimond, "Medical Education and Care in People's Republic of China," *Journal of American Medical Association*, 218 (1971): 1552-57.

20. Horn, *Away with All Pests*, pp. 78-80.

21. Wu Ying-kai, "Progress of Surgery in China," *Chinese Medical Journal* 84 (1965): 351-61.

22. Horn, *Away with All Pests*, pp. 79-80.

23. Chow Ying-ching et al., "The Integration of Modern and Traditional Chinese Medicine in the Treatment of Fractures. IV: Treatment of Colles' Fractures," *Chinese Medical Journal* 83 (1964): 425-29.

24. Peking Acupunctural Anesthesia Coordinating Group, "The Principle of Acupunctural Anesthesia." *Peking Review* 15, nos. 7-8 (1972): 17-20.

25. Heinrich Wallnöfer and Anna von Rottauscher, *Chinese Folk Medicine* (New York: Crown Publishers, 1965): pp. 125-26.

26. Ibid., p. 144.

27. Palos, *The Chinese Art*, pp. 152-60.

28. Ibid., pp. 162-63.

29. Pierre Huard and Ming Wong, *Chinese Medicine* (London: World University Library, 1968): pp. 223-29.

30. Department of Acupunctural Anesthesia of the Peking Tuberculosis Research Institute, "How Thoracic Operations Are Done under Acupunctural Anesthesia." *Peking Review* 15, nos. 7-8 (1972): 20.

31. Palos, *The Chinese Art*, p. 170.

32. Wallnöfer and von Rottauscher, *Chinese Folk Medicine*, pp. 125-44.

33. Palos, *The Chinese Art*, p. 40.

34. E. Grey Dimond, "Acupuncture Anesthesia: Western Medicine and Chinese Traditional Medicine," *Journal of the American Medical Association* 218 (1971): 1558-63.

35. Peking Acupunctural Group, "The Principle of Acupunctural Anesthesia."

36. Ibid.

37. *Medical Workers Serving the People Wholeheartedly* (Peking: Foreign Languages Press, 1971): p. 46.

38. "What Is the Right Attitude to Take in Writing Medical Articles," *Kiangsu Journal of Chinese Traditional Medicine* no. 12 (December 1964), trans. by Joint Publications Research Service, no. 43414 (November 22, 1967).

39. Ch'en Han-wei, "On the Problem of Infection Arising from Acupuncture," *Kwangtung Medical Journal—Chinese Traditional Medicine* no. 4 (July 1965): 39-40, trans. by Joint Publication Research Service, no. 43815 (December 22, 1967).

40. Peking Acupunctural Group, "The Principle of Acupunctural Anesthesia."

41. "Treating Acute Abdominal Cases without Operations," *Peking Review* 14, no. 50 (1971): 31.

42. Chen Wen-chieh and Ha Hsien-wen, "Medical and Health Work in New China." (Unpublished talk given by two Chinese physicians during a visit to Canada in November 1971.)

43. "China Creates Acupunctural Anesthesia."

44. Dimond, "Acupuncture Anesthesia."

45. Department of Acupunctural Anesthesia, "How Thoracic Operations Are Done."

46. Peking Acupunctural Group, "The Principle of Acupunctural Anesthesia."

47. Ibid.

48. Ibid.

49. Sheila Ostrander and Lynn Schroeder, "Psychic Enigmas and Energies in the U.S.S.R.," *Psychic* (May-June 1971): 9-13.

50. H. Jack Geiger, "How Acupuncture Anesthetized: The Chinese Explanation," *Medical World News* 14, no. 2 (1973): 51-61.

51. Ronald Melzack and Patrick D. Wall, "Pain Mechanisms: A Theory," *Science* 150 (1965): 971-79.

52. Ronald Melzack, "How Acupuncture Works: A Sophisticated Western Theory Takes the Mystery Out," *Psychology Today* 7, no. 6 (June 1973): 28-35.

53. Bernard Straus, "Acupuncture—A Powerful Placebo," *Medical Tribune* (September 15, 1971).

54. Boyce Rensberger, "U.S. Doctors Are Skeptical of Acupuncture in Treatment of Purely Physical Diseases," *The New York Times* (October 7, 1971).

55. Stephen M. Krane, "Action of Salicylates," *The New England Journal of Medicine* 286 (1972): 317-18.

VII. The Treatment
of Mental Illness

A REVIEW of mental health facilities in China is a particularly difficult task, since many of the premises involved in psychiatric care differ greatly from those in the West. For those of us trained in Freudian thinking the task involves putting our assumptions to one side, for a time, and examining a very different view of man and his psyche. Of crucial importance in the Chinese view of man is the belief in his ability to change, given a sympathetic environment and "education and reeducation." Underlying this view, in fact running through all activities in the society, is politics. As our hosts frequently told us, "We put politics in command." And as we shall see, politics is in command in the area of mental health.

The organization of Chinese society today must be considered in any discussion of mental health. It seems to be a society of great consensus; similar customs and mores apply to vast numbers of the population. Basic needs such as food, clothing, housing, jobs, education, and medical care are now guaranteed to essentially the entire population, albeit at a minimal level. No one is left to fend for himself; the population both in the cities and in the countryside is divided into small units characterized by self-reliance and mutual help. While the individual is expected to work hard and participate extensively in local affairs, he is also cared for by his family, neighbors, or associates at work when he is in need of such care. In addition there is apparently little tolerance of asocial or antisocial behavior, and great pressure is undoubtedly applied to assure conformity to the approved way of life.

Our view of Chinese mental health services was extremely limited. In 1971 we visited the psychiatric department of the

Peking Third Hospital and the Shanghai Mental Hospital, and talked with doctors, nurses, and members of the revolutionary committees of both hospitals at some length. In addition, we were able to gather general information on the structure of Chinese society and its relationship to mental health from our hosts in the Chinese Medical Association. In 1972 we talked at length with Dr. Wu Chen-i, professor in the Department of Psychiatry, Peking Medical College, and Dr. Shen Yu-chun, director of the department. They further elucidated some of the principles of treating mental illness, particularly the concept of "revolutionary optimism."

THE "BITTER PAST"

Long before Western psychiatric theories entered Chinese medical thinking there were two divergent streams of thought that explained mental illness: the philosophical or medical approach, and folk beliefs and folk medical practices. Both theories have had great impact on modern Chinese psychiatric thinking.

To look at the philosophical or medical body of thought first, ancient Chinese medical writings attributed all disease, including mental illness, to an imbalance of two forces: the *yin* and the *yang*. According to Ilza Veith, "These two forces which stand for the negative and the positive, the dark and the white, the moon and the sun, the noxious and the beneficial, also denote the female and male elements, both of which are present in man and woman alike. Disease arises when the proportions of the two elements begin to vary from the normal." [1] The imbalance between the *yin* and the *yang* was thought to be caused by deviation from the *tao,* the "way," which provided the guide for all morality and human conduct. The *tao* can be further thought of as being an "ethical superstructure" that "provided for all eventualities in life and for all essential types of interpersonal relationships." [2] Once transgression against this ethical superstructure occurred, return to health was through a return to *tao.*

While there was no supernatural element in the philosophical or medical explanation, the popular or folk beliefs about the

origins of mental illness were based almost entirely on supernatural causes. And while the believers in *tao* saw the mind and
the body as indivisible, popular belief considered the mind and
the body as separate entities. Spirits and demons were thought
from earliest times to be responsible for many of the ills that
befell man. Spirits were thought to be everywhere,

> . . . in the water, the caves, the trees, and graves, they lurked in
> the soil and under rocks. They swarmed about the homes of men
> in populated as well as in isolated regions and, according to many
> tales, their favorite abodes were the privies, where man is alone
> and helpless and flight difficult.[3]

Once a demon or spirit entered a person and made him ill
it needed to be exorcised. The first exorcists were members of a
priesthood called *wu,* which to the present day has the meaning
of wizard, witch, expeller of demons. *Wu* is first encountered
in the *Rites of the Chou Dynasty* (1122–255 B.C.), and it came
eventually to be synonymous with the word for physician, *wu-i*
meaning "magical physician."[4] The *wu,* who might be either
male or female, was thought to be able to cure because he had
a greater proportion of *yang* than ordinary people. To exorcise
the spirit or demon that had entered the sick person, the *wu*
might put him into a deep sleep, might dance around him, and
was likely to inflict wounds upon himself as a method of cure.

Among the spirits that might enter a person, those of the
dead were greatly feared, especially of people who had not had
proper funeral observances or who had died through violence.
It was thought that the spirits of the dead could steal the souls
of the living while they were asleep and their souls were occupied
with dreams. Since the spirits of the dead were thought to be so
powerful, much of the work of the medical priests was in attempting to appease their hostility. One group of spirits were thought
to be more powerful than the others—the *t'ien ku,* otherwise
known as "celestial dog." They were thought to be able to speak
to their victims, to inflict amnesia upon them, and to particularly
disturb young boys.

In the folklore of both China and Japan the fox was also
thought to have great powers. The fox was believed to be so

powerful that it could not only bring on mental disease but could impersonate those who could cure mental illness, thereby causing massive confusion. During the Han dynasty and the Han period of literature (206 B.C.–A.D. 280) the fear of foxes was widespread.[5] The fox also seems to have played a great role in sexual seductions and assaults, sometimes occupying the bodies of young women, sometimes of men. The following passage from the *Hsuan-chung-chi*, written in the first few centuries A.D., demonstrates the power the fox was thought to have:

> When a fox is fifty years old, it becomes a beautiful female . . . or a grown-up man who has sexual intercourse with women. Such beings are able to know things occurring at more than a thousand miles distant; they can poison men by sorcery, or possess them and bewilder them, so that they lose their memory and knowledge. And when a fox is a thousand years old, it penetrates to heaven and becomes a Celestial Fox.[6]

Since the mentally ill person was thought to be possessed by a spirit or demon or fox, the onset of illness was swift; the cure might be equally sudden for the *wu*, by his ministrations, could exorcise the demon quickly. Swift exorcism led to a belief in the curability of mental illness that seems to have been carried through to the present. The theory of possession by demons also leads logically to the attachment of no blame to the patient himself, thereby reducing the stigma attached to mental illness.

Other popular beliefs about the origin of mental illness were that one might have been guilty of a misdeed in one's previous life; that one's ancestors might have offended the gods who were now punishing the offspring; that the god of the wind was using the insane man's home as a temporary residence, and that his spirit was living in the ill person's body; that some organ inside the body was deformed or had lost its function; or that the circulation of blood within the ill person was running in the opposite direction from that of the normal person. It was felt that mental control was through the heart, and that if the heart lost control the body was then without direction."[7]

These were some of the prevalent beliefs of the causes of mental illness when the first mental hospital was opened in Canton in 1897. Although it started with only thirty beds and increased in size to 500 beds it was closed in the 1930s.[8] The first academic division of neurology was established at Peking Union Medical College in 1921, the year it was founded, as part of the Department of Medicine. A Department of Psychiatry and Neurology was established at PUMC in 1932. The growth of psychiatry and neurology in China up to 1949 was very slow, however; in 1948 there were only about 1,000 beds for psychiatric patients in all of China.[9]

In 1949 there were four psychiatric hospitals, one each in Peking, Shanghai, Canton, and Nanking; patients were often cruelly treated, bound to their beds, and given very little psychiatric care.[10] By the 1930s and 1940s most people suffering from mental illness were still being kept at home with their families; if they were found in the street doing anything wrong they might be "thrown into prison and treated as if they are criminals. If they are harmless and wander in the streets, they are mocked and laughed at and are often stoned." [11]

Estimates of the incidence of mental disease in China in the mid-1930s range from as low as 1:1,000 population, or 400,000 mentally ill people, to 1:400, or 1–1.25 million people.[12] The widespread poverty, violence, and starvation, and the brutalizing effect these conditions had on family life provided fertile ground for mental illness. The cruelty to which a woman was subjected —being sold into marriage at an early age, having to serve her husband's family, being brutally treated by her husband and particularly by her mother-in-law, and bearing many children most of whom might well die—drove many women to suicide and others undoubtedly to mental illness.

Prior to 1949 venereal disease was an important cause of mental illness. The earliest estimates of the existence of prostitution in China are from the Chou dynasty in 650 B.C. Venereal disease appears to have been introduced during the Ming dynasty, A.D. 1368–1644, starting in Kwangtung Province and spreading north.[13] At the time of Liberation the prevalence of syphilis was said to be 5 per cent in the cities and as high as 10 per cent in the national minority areas.[14] Although there was some effort to control and treat venereal disease, medical techniques were hindered by the popular belief that it was a logical punishment for misdeeds.[15]

Another major cause of mental illness prior to 1949 was drug addiction. It has been estimated that in the mid-1930s [16] there were 300,000 addicts in Peking alone. In 1935 the Nationalist government launched a six-year program aimed at "the total suppression of the chronic use of morphine and heroin" within two years, and opium within six years. Compulsory treatment was inaugurated, consisting of two to three weeks of hospitalization, followed by hard labor to build up the addict's physical condition. There was a large percentage of relapses, however, and in 1937 addicts began to receive severe punishments; some recidivists were executed and others sent to prison.[17]

FROM LIBERATION TO CULTURAL REVOLUTION

Between 1949 and 1965 the government put great stress on medical care. In 1952, when the Chinese Society of Neurology and Psychiatry was established in affiliation with the Chinese Medical Association in Peking, there were only 100 neuropsychiatrists in China; by 1967 this figure had risen to 436.

By 1957 the number of psychiatric beds had been increased to 20,000, and new methods of treating mentally ill patients had been introduced. Isolation and the binding of patients were prohibited and work therapy was introduced. Before the Cultural Revolution all the medical schools had courses in psychiatry, and neuropsychiatric research was carried on widely. From 1958 through 1961 electroencephalographic research was conducted, as was research on schizophrenia.[18] Psychiatric services spread at an even greater rate in the late 1950s and early 1960s. There have been reports of treatment of mental illnesses in the autonomous region of Inner Mongolia and in Urumchi, the center of the Sinkiang Uighur autonomous region.[19]

Before the Cultural Revolution traditional medicine—including acupuncture, ignipuncture, breathing exercises, and the use of herb medicine—and Western medicine were used in the treatment of mental disease. (Acupuncture will be dealt with in

greater detail later in this chapter.) Ignipuncture is "treatment
by means of thermal excitation through various methods of cautery
and burning at empirically determined points of the body." [20]
Sometimes acupuncture and ignipuncture were combined in a
course of treatment called *chen chu,* which dates back 2,000 years
in the treatment of psychoses, neuroses, and headaches. The
breathing exercises were similar to those used by Buddhist monks,
and therapeutic results were obtained after regular use of the
exercises, morning and evening, for several months.[21]

THE CURRENT SCENE

Since the Cultural Revolution there has been increased
emphasis in all branches of medicine on combining the techniques
of traditional and Western medicine. While the Chinese had
been doing so in other branches of medical care since 1949,
from the time of Liberation until 1965 the psychiatric sphere
seems to have concentrated more on Western methods of treatment and to have neglected traditional techniques. Using the
slogan "Let the past serve the present and let the foreign serve
China," since the Cultural Revolution, Western-trained doctors
have been revamping their psychiatric services to include traditional methods and political techniques adopted by the society at
large.

As with all other institutions, in 1971 psychiatric hospitals
were run by revolutionary committees consisting of the usual
three-in-one combination: the People's Liberation Army, cadres
(political workers), and members of the mass. The mass is composed of those people who work in any institution; in a mental
hospital it consists of doctors, nurses, auxiliary workers, and
cleaning help. The revolutionary committees often include the
other three-in-one combination of aged, middle-aged, and young
people. The revolutionary committee at the Shanghai Mental
Hospital, which was founded in 1958, is made up of fifteen
members, eleven men and four women. The hospital has thirteen
wards, five for women and eight for men, with a total of 916
beds. The staff includes sixty-one doctors and 169 nurses.

The methods currently being used to treat mental illness are collective help, self-reliance, drug therapy, acupuncture, "heart-to-heart talks," follow-up care, community ethos, productive labor, the teachings of Chairman Mao Tse-tung, and "revolutionary optimism."

Collective Help. With the participation of members of the People's Liberation Army in the administration of hospitals since the Cultural Revolution, some psychiatric hospitals are using the army model of organization, dividing the patients on the wards into groups so that they can become a "collective fighting group instead of a ward." Within these "fighting groups" the patients who are getting better are paired with newer and sicker patients so that they can help each other with "mutual love and mutual help."

Self-Reliance. The patients themselves are encouraged to investigate their own disease, to examine their symptoms, and to understand their treatment. They are encouraged to study themselves in order to recognize their condition and to prevent a relapse.

Drug Therapy. Seriously ill patients are given "thorazine" (chlorpromazine), though evidently in smaller doses than before the Cultural Revolution. Insulin shock and electric shock therapy have been eliminated since the Cultural Revolution.

Acupuncture. Three kinds of acupuncture are used for certain forms of schizophrenia: (1) Acupuncture needles placed in the temples, or behind or in front of the ears, hooked up to a battery box for three to five minutes at a time, once or twice a day, for a forty- to forty-five day course; (2) acupuncture of the ear; and (3) acupuncture of the legs and the arms for relief of excitement, catatonia, and depression; this treatment is generally given for fifteen to twenty minutes, three times a day.

"Heart-to-Heart Talks." A psychiatrist meets with patients individually or in small groups at regular intervals to discuss their problems and to help them understand their illness more completely. We were told that the most important form of treatment is the relationship between the psychiatrist and the patient.

Follow-Up Care. After the patient is discharged he is followed up, first, every two weeks, and then monthly, in the out-

patient department. Sometimes a doctor or a nurse on the staff
of the hospital will make a home visit. Before discharge a doctor
will visit the patient's place of work to make sure that he is
returning to a job that is best for his mental health. Although the
patient's job has been kept for him pending his return, it may
be that another task within his work unit would better suit his
mental health needs. Often the patient is kept on chlorpromazine
after discharge, but on a smaller dosage.

Community Ethos. In 1971 we were told that every neighborhood, both urban and rural, is organized under the direction of a
committee made up of members of the People's Liberation Army,
cadres, and the mass—the people who live in the neighborhood.
The elected members of the neighborhood committee provide
social services, mediate disputes, do marital counseling, and in
general look after the residents of the community. When a patient
is about to be discharged from a mental hospital he becomes the
"special concern" of his neighborhood committee as well as of his
family and friends; this community concern plus the assurance of
his job and family waiting for him help ease the transition from
hospital to community.

Productive Labor. As in the larger society, where all members
are encouraged to do productive labor, hospital patients are also
encouraged to do what we in the West would call occupational
therapy. Patients were seen folding bandages and preparing medications for the outpatient department, and doing work for a local
factory, such as making covers for toothpaste tubes. The factory
pays the hospital for the patients' work and this income is used
to provide them with special services.

The Teachings of Chairman Mao. Running through this
entire gamut of treatment techniques is the philosophy of Chairman Mao. Inspired by his maxim, "Heal the wounded and rescue
the dead," patients and hospital workers alike study his writings:
"On Practice," "On Contradiction," "Where Do Correct Ideas
Come From?," and the "Three Constantly-Read Articles"—"Serve
the People," "In Memory of Norman Bethune," and "The Foolish
Old Man Who Removed the Mountains." Patients are organized
into groups to study these writings daily and are encouraged

through them to understand "objective reality," rather than function on the basis of "subjective thinking." They "arm their minds with Chairman Mao's Thought during their stay in the hospital in order to fight their disease."

"Revolutionary Optimism." A psychiatric patient is encouraged to feel that he is part of a force greater than himself, that of the revolution. He is urged to believe that the revolution will be victorious and that "no matter what the difficulties, he will have a bright future." It is important for the patient to receive treatment and to overcome his disease not only for his own sake, but for the sake of the revolution. Revolutionary optimism gives the patient the "encouragemement and the confidence to conquer his disease."

THE PATIENT

In the psychiatric department of the Third Teaching Hospital of the Peking Medical College, which has two wards, one for men and one for women, with ninety beds, we visited the patients' club where there were about fifty patients wearing red pajamas and red and white striped robes. Four of the patients gathered around a table to tell us and the other patients, "How I used Chairman Mao's Thought to conquer difficulties." The first to speak was a thirty-two-year-old man with the diagnosis of paranoid schizophrenia who had been in the hospital for three months:

> At the time of the last spring festival I had a quarrel with my wife. She said she wanted to divorce me and I was surprised. I returned to work but I was suspicious of my wife and kept thinking that she would divorce me. At that time my wife was not working in Peking and I asked to have her transferred to Peking and asked her to send my letters back. We quarrelled a lot because I insisted that she wanted to divorce me and she said that she did not.
>
> During my early period of admission to the hospital I did not know that I had mental trouble. Gradually I recognized that something was wrong in my mentality and I gradually recognized that I had to make a class analysis of the causes of my disease in order to facilitate treatment and prevention.
>
> My trouble was that I had subjective thinking which was not

objectively correct. My wife had not written letters wanting to divorce me; my wife actually loves me. My subjective thinking was divorced from the practical condition and my disease was caused by my method of thinking. I was concerned with the individual person; I was self-interested. I haven't put revolutionary interests in the first place, but if I can put the public interest first and my own interest second I can solve the contradictions and my mind will be in the correct way. From now on I will study Chairman Mao and apply his writings.

The next patient who spoke was a woman in her twenties:

I was a graduate of junior middle school and in 1969 was sent out to work in an outlying province. I was admitted five months ago to this hospital but I am getting alright now. My main trouble is auditory hallucinations. I hear something in my ear saying, "What is below your pillow?" I found old magazines on the subject of a biological radio apparatus and I came to the ridiculous conclusion that a special agent is investigating me by means of this biological radio apparatus. I became agitated and heard loud speeches in my mind which gave me a very bad headache. During the midst of my torture I was sent to the hospital and received medication. My headache is much better but I still have hallucinations.

The doctors organized a study class of Chairman Mao's works and I joined the class and studied the five works. I studied my hallucinations and gradually recognized that they were nonexistent. I found that investigation is like a pregnancy, and solving problems is like delivering a baby. As I investigated my problem I gradually recognized that the biological radio was nonexistent. Now I still have some hallucinations but after ten minutes I recognize that they are not real. Now whenever I have hallucinations, I study the works of Chairman Mao and attract [sic] my mind and my heart so I will get rid of my trouble.

My treatments consist of acupuncture, medicine, herb medicine, and study. Also I am considering what happens in the whole world. I talk with doctors and patients; I do physical exercises; I have not completely recovered yet but I have faith I will get better and will win the struggle.

The last patient,* a young woman who was a middle school graduate with a diagnosis of schizophrenia, had been hospitalized

_____
* The third patient's presentation is given in Chapter IV (see page 108).

for two months but had been discharged when her condition improved. She returns periodically for a checkup and on the morning we visited the ward she had been invited back to talk with the new patients and to help teach them how to arm themselves with Chairman Mao's Thought. She was dressed in street clothes and told us the following story:

I was a senior middle school graduate in 1967 but my health was not good at that time. I had heart trouble and arthritis and was not sent out to work like my classmates. Last April I was called to have a discussion with regard to my work and I got my mental trouble at that time.

I was born in the new society and therefore have not suffered as people did in the old society. I was educated for more than ten years and then rested at home for two years due to my illnesses. Thus I was divorced for twelve years from practice, class struggle, and revolutionary experience. I was a "hot-house flower."

I knew that sick people were kept in Peking and not sent out to remote areas and I thought day and night about where I would work. I had a fixed opinion that I had to work here in Peking, not elsewhere. I didn't want to eat and I didn't want to drink. I dreamt of being a People's Liberation Army woman at that time and had suspicions and fantastic ideas. Whenever I saw a member of the PLA or a PLA car I thought it would take me to the People's Liberation Army.

During my early period of admission I could not manage myself. I threw pillows through windows and had to be fed. I thought I was going to be poisoned here and that I had to struggle against the hospital. When other patients sang army songs I thought the PLA was here already. Gradually I realized that the doctors and nurses were here to serve the patient. They washed my hair and clothing and I gradually realized that this is a hospital. I then participated in a study group and studied the "Three Constantly-Read Articles" for two weeks. I learned that my hallucinations and suspicions were not real and found that studying in a study class was a good way to solve one's problems. I understood that one has to have knowledge before experience and then try to understand objective reality.

When a member of the PLA visited the hospital I thought it was for me and I raised the issue in my study group. The doctors told me it was just a visit by that member and it was not for me and I believed them.

I was discharged over three months ago and although my new

job was supposed to be arranged July 1, it has not been arranged yet. But I now have full faith in the Communist Party and the government and know that they will arrange a job for me later on. Until then I will continue to take my medicine and have close contact with the medical people in this hospital.

The doctors at the Shanghai Mental Hospital consider schizophrenia to be the most common diagnosis—over 50 per cent of their patients are schizophrenics. Paranoia is believed to be the most common form of schizophrenia; depression, catatonia, and postpartum depression are relatively rare. The suicide rate is said to be quite low.

The hospital also admits a small percentage of patients who have physical illnesses with psychiatric complications, such as disturbed liver function, epilepsy, and heart disease. Both the Shanghai Mental Hospital and the psychiatric ward of the Third Teaching Hospital in Peking reported that the most common age of onset of mental illness is from twenty to thirty years of age. This corroborates findings in the 1930s that revealed that onset of mental illness in 40 per cent of the patients in one study occurred between ages twenty to thirty.[22]

In a study of a group of 2,000 schizophrenics done in the late 1950s, it was found that 50 per cent were between the ages of twenty-one and thirty; 1.3 per cent were under fifteen years of age; and over 7 per cent were over forty. More than 46 per cent of these schizophrenics were paranoid, 24 per cent were "unclassified," 15 per cent hebephrenic, and 11 per cent catatonic.[23]

THE PERSONNEL

Before the Cultural Revolution most psychiatrists attended medical school for five years and, during the final year, interned in a department of psychiatry in a teaching hospital specializing in psychiatry, internal medicine, and neurology. They would then remain in a hospital psychiatric department continuing their studies by doing "practical work," making rounds, attending lectures, and treating patients under the supervision of residents. A psychiatrist was considered trained when the senior doctors in his department felt he was adequately prepared; there was no examination or fixed period of study. Since medical schools have only recently reopened following the Cultural Revolution, a new pattern has yet to be established. The number of women in psychiatry at the present time was thought to be over 50 per cent.

Nurses are trained under the same basic principles. Again, before the Cultural Revolution they attended nursing school and received some psychiatric training. They then had on-the-job practical training in a psychiatric ward to which they were assigned and attended some lectures.

The works of Freud have not been used in the study of psychiatry since 1949; the works of Pavlov have been studied, however, particularly during the period of Russian influence, but our hosts told us that without "considerable environmental and class struggle" the application of Pavlov's theories will not be effective.

HOSPITAL LIFE

At the Shanghai Mental Hospital we attended a Mao Tse-tung study class that met from 2:00 to 3:30 every afternoon for two weeks. Eleven patients dressed in brown uniforms sat around a table with a member of the PLA and a member of a Mao Tse-tung propaganda team who works in the hospital and takes part in the class when he is free. A health worker who is in charge of the patients' study group in this ward was also present. Two of the patients around the table were wearing red armbands to indicate that they were on duty. Their main task is to propagandize Mao's Thought when new patients come into their ward; they tell them their own experiences and help them get used to their new surroundings. The patients on duty rotate so that everyone in the ward has a chance to perform these tasks.

The group studied the "Third Constantly Read Article," "The Foolish Old Man Who Removed the Mountains," and one patient told the parable of an old man who had a mountain on his property. When he and his sons started to remove it with shovels his neighbors scoffed at him, but he insisted that if his sons and his sons' sons worked to remove the mountain it could be done. The patient explained that they should all learn the

170

spirit of the parable and put it into practice in order to strengthen their will and conquer their illness.

Patients live two, four, eight, or sixteen to a room, depending on the severity of their condition. There were a few rooms with a single patient and some of these were locked. The rooms were furnished very simply with beds, bureaus, and posters or slogans on the walls. The patients make their beds and sweep the floors with the help of the health workers. The daily schedule posted on one wall reads as follows:

5:00-5:30 A.M.		Get up and make beds
5:30-6:00 "		Breakfast
6:00-7:30 "		Occupational therapy
6:30-7:00 " (Friday)		Military training
7:30-8:30 "		Study Chairman Mao's work
8:30-10:00 " (Monday, Wednesday, Friday)		Heart-to-heart talks
8:30-10:00 " (Tuesday, Thursday, Saturday)		Study class
10:00-10:30 "		Treatment
10:30-11:30 "		Lunch, free time
12:00-1:30 P.M.		Nap
1:30-2:00 "		News
2:30-3:30 "		Study class
3:30-4:15 " (Monday, Wednesday, Friday)		Physical activities
3:30-6:30 " (Tuesday, Thursday, Saturday)		Visits from relatives
4:30 p.m.		Supper
Evening		Television
9:30 p.m.		Bed

Exhortatory messages were also up on the walls. Lin Piao's quotations read: "Read Chairman Mao's works. Listen to Chairman Mao. Work according to Chairman Mao's teachings. Act as good fighters for Chairman Mao." In another room of the

Shanghai Mental Hospital a poster on the wall was entitled, "How to Prevent Disease Relapse." The first two items read:

1. Mental disease is curable.
2. Being a psychiatric patient you still have to study Chairman Mao's works hard.

The third point dealt with acupuncture; the fourth point read: "Sometimes you will have symptoms. Don't worry. If you get treatment right away relapse can be avoided."

In the patients' activity room they were playing Chinese chess and ping-pong, doing occupational therapy, and reading small comic-like books. A loudspeaker was playing a lively song from a modern revolutionary opera. Slogans hung across the room stated: "Hold High the Red Banner of Mao's Thought," and "Warmly Celebrate the Founding of the People's Republic of China." Those patients who are doing particularly well in their "struggle against their illness" have short essays written about them by their doctors and other patients and these too are posted on the wall. Also posted is a list of the patients who are paired together to help each other, the sicker with the healthier.

The average length of hospitalization in the Shanghai Mental Hospital is seventy days. The doctors told us that before the Cultural Revolution the relapse rate of schizophrenics was a problem—40 per cent of the patients were likely to have two or three admissions. Relapse is interpreted to mean the need for readmission or for outpatient treatment. Currently the emphasis is on reeducation, "right before the patients are discharged, on how to deal with the environment and contradictions within the environment." The doctors have been conducting follow-up studies on the relapse rate and have found that in one ward that was studied for a year 18.3 per cent of the patients suffered relapses. In a one-year study of thirty-seven patients on another ward, they found one relapsed patient who was treated both at home and in the outpatient department. The psychiatrists said that the most important factor mitigating against a high relapse rate is the Mao study class, "to arm them with Mao's Thought to better deal with the environment."

Acupuncture is considered a major method of treatment in the lowering of the relapse rate. The doctors at the Shanghai Mental Hospital have divided the criteria for success of acupuncture treatment into four levels: (1) Cured—disappearance of symptoms, with the patient "managing everything by his own mentality"; (2) much improved—disappearance of symptoms with the patient "mostly managing by his own mentality"; (3) improved—with some remaining symptoms; and (4) unimproved. They recently conducted a one-year study of 157 cases of schizophrenia and found that 74.3 per cent were cured or much improved; 97.4 per cent fell in the first three categories, that is, cured, much improved, and improved. Without acupuncture treatment there is a 70 per cent relapse rate.

Because of recent disclosures of the political use of psychiatry in the Soviet Union, the process of psychiatric hospitalization seems an important one to understand. The doctors on the psychiatric ward of the Third Teaching Hospital in Peking said that hospitalization is nearly always through the persuasion of relatives, friends, and colleagues at work. Admission to the hospital is generally a joint effort by the patient's family and the authorities of the unit in which he works, who usually all agree on the need for hospitalization. Occasionally commitment is by force, but this is said to be exceptional.

After admission, the patient may need to be persuaded by the personnel to remain and to receive treatment. The technique of new patients being welcomed by the older patients who help them to adjust was considered important in this beginning phase of hospitalization. As the patient recovers slightly sometimes he must be persuaded to stay until he is thoroughly improved. The doctors maintain that a patient never leaves the hospital against their advice because the physicians have obtained the cooperation of members of the revolutionary committee where the patient works and of his family. They stressed that the patient respects the opinions of the authorities of his work unit, and if the doctor, the patient's family, and the revolutionary committee all agree, he is likely to abide by their decision.

BASIC PRINCIPLES OF TREATMENT

The treatment of mental illness in the People's Republic of China is a process involving multiple techniques: traditional and Western medicine, group and individual relationships, professional and nonprofessional care, mutual help and self-reliance, and hospital and community involvement.

Since the Cultural Revolution, new models of organizing patients in mental hospitals to "raise the patient's initiative to fight his disease" are being tried extensively. The writing and thinking of Mao Tse-tung underlies all of these efforts.

Several basic characteristics of Chinese society are critical to the handling of mental illness:

1. The society is extraordinarily cohesive, and the effects of this cohesion have not begun to be explored with regard to the incidence and treatment of mental illness.

2. The organization of the society into small groups in which mutual help and local participation are emphasized must be regarded both as an effort at preventive mental health and as an adjunct to the treatment of mental patients.

3. The belief in the malleability and perfectability of man through "education and reeducation" is the foundation on which many of the new techniques, such as Mao Tse-tung study groups, are based.

4. Although the Chinese are attempting to fashion their own brand of mental health services through using their social structure and their traditional medicine, they do incorporate Western techniques such as drug therapy when they feel they are useful.

Throughout the Chinese medical care system, as well as in other facets of life, their pragmatism and willingness to experiment are highly evident. Thus the treatment of mental illness in China is likely to be a changing picture that we in the West would do well to observe.

NOTES

1. Ilza Veith, "Psychiatric Thought in Chinese Medicine," *Journal of the History of Medicine and Allied Sciences* 10 (1955): 261-68.
2. Ibid.

3. Idem, "The Supernatural in Far Eastern Concepts of Mental Disease," *Bulletin of the History of Medicine* 37 (1963): 139-55.

4. Ibid.

5. Ibid.

6. Ibid.

7. Herbert Day Lamson, *Social Pathology in China* (Shanghai: The Commercial Press, 1935): pp. 415-16.

8. Veith, "Psychiatric Thought in Chinese Medicine."

9. J. Cerny, "Chinese Psychiatry," *International Journal of Psychiatry* 1 (1965): 229-38.

10. Ibid.

11. Lamson, *Social Pathology in China*, p. 416.

12. Ibid., p. 410.

13. Ibid., pp. 109-12.

14. George Hatem, "With Mao Tse-tung's Thought as the Compass for Action in the Control of Venereal Diseases in China," *China's Medicine* no. 10 (October 1966): 52-68.

15. Lamson, *Social Pathology in China*, p. 366.

16. R. S. Lyman, V. Maeker, and P. Liang, eds., *Neuropsychiatry in China* (Peking: Henri Vetch, 1939): p. 234.

17. Ibid., p. 233.

18. Cerny, "Chinese Psychiatry."

19. Ibid.

20. Ibid.

21. Ibid.

22. Lamson, *Social Pathology in China*, p. 411.

23. Cerny, "Chinese Psychiatry."

VIII. Health Administration and Research

A S was discussed in Chapter I, China's Ministry of Health, which had played an important policy-making role from 1949 to 1965, was severely criticized and dismantled during the Cultural Revolution. The minister of health, Chien Hsin-chung, was removed in 1967.[1] During our 1971 visit we were told that the ministry was still undergoing "struggle, criticism, and transformation," and, despite our request to do so, we were given no opportunity to speak with anyone representing the ministry or even the bureaus of public health at the provincial or local levels.

The situation had changed markedly by the time of our visit in 1972. Hsieh Hua, a military physician who had served in the People's Liberation Army and who had been introduced to us in 1971 as the "responsible member" of the Chinese Medical Association (CMA), was introduced in 1972 in both that role and as a "leading member" of the Ministry of Health. The first announcement in English of this title for Hsieh Hua was in a statement by *Hsinhua* (New China News Agency) that a visiting delegation had met with him in July 1972. Others identified to us in 1972 as members of the Ministry of Health were Chen Jen-hung and Yen Chuan. Hsu Shou-jen, an administrator who accompanied us through our 1971 visit in his capacity as "secretary-general of the CMA," was introduced in 1972 as deputy secretary-general of the association and as a member of the ministry. In short, it appears that the Ministry of Health and the CMA are currently closely intertwined and in some ways inseparable.

Similar relationships are found at more local levels. In 1971

175

Hong Ming-gui, also a former military physician, was introduced
as the responsible member of the Shanghai branch of the CMA;
in 1972 he was in addition identified as the leading member of the
Shanghai Bureau of Public Health.

In 1972 it became possible for us to talk at length with members of the bureaus of public health of Peking and of Shanghai.
The role of the Shanghai bureau provides an example of the
way public health administration is now functioning, and its relationship with other community services. There are more than
thirty bureaus in the city, each related to a department or ministry in the national government. In addition to public health, the
Shanghai bureaus include education, publications, motion pic-
tures, athletics, civil affairs, labor, public safety, public utilities,
postal and telegraph, and agriculture. Shanghai is governed by
a revolutionary committee of 150 members; some, but not all,
bureau chiefs are members of the committee; Dr. Hong, the chief
of the Bureau of Public Health, is a member.

There are six departments in the Bureau of Public Health:
(1) Curative medicine, pharmacy, hygiene, and public health,
which has jurisdiction over hospitals, maternal and child health,
middle medical schools, occupational hygiene, communicable disease, pharmacies, and barefoot doctors; (2) medical research; (3)
emergency medical care; (4) administration; (5) finance; and (6)
personnel. The total staff of the bureau is approximately 120,
but some of its work is carried out through the Shanghai branch
of the CMA which employs sixty people.

The Municipal Public Health Station, operated by the Department of Curative Medicine, Pharmacy, Hygiene, and Public
Health, employs 300 to 400 people, most of whom are assigned
to district and county stations. They have responsibility for
epidemiology, sanitation, school health, and nutrition. There is
also a Municipal Occupational Health Station with 200 inpatient
beds, and a station in each district charged specifically with over-
seeing BCG vaccinations against tuberculosis. Each district has a
dental station, often located inside the district hospital. There
are mental health stations in each district as well as in a few
counties.

Among the proudest accomplishments of the Shanghai Bureau of Public Health is the cleaning up of Shanghai's environment, which is being done in collaboration with other bureaus involved. For example, Chaochiapang Creek was described as having been "a stinking stream contaminated by industrial waste," and "a source of diseases which often became epidemic among working people." In a joint effort the creek was filled in and made into a boulevard lined with trees and flowers. The effluence from the factories is now carried away by a sewage system, and the bureau has helped to develop new production methods to reduce pollutant discharge. For example, the Kwangming electroplating factory formerly used sodium cyanide and discharged 450 to 600 tons of effluence containing cyanide daily; it now uses a new electroplating technique that eliminates the need for cyanide.[2] The bureau has the power to incorporate systems for treating industrial waste into the designs of all new factories being built.

The bureau also has responsibility for maintaining statistics on Shanghai's health status. The data provided us by the bureau in 1972—the first health statistics of their type to be released since the Cultural Revolution—are presented and analyzed in Appendix E.

In general it appears that the municipal and provincial bureaus of public health have responsibility for most personal and public health services, and for nonphysician health worker education. They share responsibility for some health care with specific operating agencies, such as the railways; for physician education, with the Bureau of Education; for research, with the Academy of Medical Sciences; and for biological and pharmaceutical standards, with bureaus responsible for production. Not surprisingly, the bureaus and their departments operate through decentralized structures. Each level of government—city, municipal, district, neighborhood, resident's committee, and even group level—has a member in charge of health work who collaborates with the corresponding levels of the bureau and its units.

The post-Cultural Revolution reconstruction of the local and provincial bureaus, and of the national Ministry of Health, is of course continuing. By the end of 1972, of China's seventeen

178   SERVE THE PEOPLE

national ministries, twelve were headed by ministers; the remainder were under vice-ministers or—as in the case of the
Ministry of Health—officials called "leading" or "responsible"
persons.[3] In May 1973 Huang Shu-tse, identified as a "vice-
minister of health," headed the first delegation of the People's
Republic of China to participate in a world health assembly.[4]
And in June 1973 a Reuter's dispatch from Peking reported the
appointment of Liu Hsiang-pin as "minister of public health."[5]
Madame Liu, the widow of former Minister of Public Security
Hsieh Fu-chih, is the first woman to hold ministerial rank in
China for many years—although other women, such as Soong
Ching-ling, widow of Dr. Sun Yat-sen and sister of Madame
Chiang Kai-shek, who holds the rank of deputy chief of state,
and Chiang Ching, wife of Mao Tse-tung, who is a member of the
Standing Committee of the Communist Party Politburo, have high
leadership positions.

THE CHINESE MEDICAL ASSOCIATION

In contrast to the Ministry of Health, about which we learned
relatively little, we learned a great deal about the CMA, our
hosts during our visits. The CMA was originally established in
April 1932 through the merger of the National Medical Association of China and the China Medical Association. The latter,
founded in 1886 as the China Medical Missionary Association,
became the China Medical Association in 1925. Its first president
was J. G. Kerr, a medical missionary in Canton, and its membership was confined almost exclusively to European and American medical missionaries; it published the *China Medical Missionary Journal,* which was renamed the *China Medical Journal*
in 1907. The National Medical Association was founded in 1915
with Yen Fu-ching, dean of the Hsiang-ya (Hunan-Yale) Medical
College, as president. Its members were Chinese physicians who
had been trained in Western-style medical colleges both in China
and abroad; it published the *National Medical Journal of China.*

The merger of the two associations was based on "the im-
mense increase in the number of well-trained Chinese physicians
in all branches of medicine," and the fact that "the initiative and

leadership of medical practice has passed to the Chinese." The editorial in the *Chinese Medical Journal,* the English-language journal formed by the merger of the *China Medical Journal* and the *National Medical Journal of China,* announcing the merger stated that the medical missionaries "particularly welcomed this advance, for part of their task in China had been to prepare the way for the sons of the soil to develop their own medical work and thus lead their own people." [6]

The published aims of the new association, with "a membership of over 1,500 of whom about one-half are foreign colleagues," were:

1. To bring into one compact organization all duly qualified and scientifically trained physicians;
2. To extend medical knowledge and advance medical science;
3. To uphold the standards of medical education;
4. To maintain the high ethical standards of the medical profession, to safeguard its material interests, and to promote friendly relations among its members;
5. To cooperate with other medical societies and agencies;
6. To issue the *Chinese Medical Journal.*

The Japanese occupation of the major urban areas of China's east coast obviously led to great problems in the functioning of the CMA. Its general secretary during that period was Szeming Sze, who was also the editor of the *Chinese Medical Journal.* In a 1943 report published by the CMA in Washington, D.C., Sze stated that the CMA had a membership of 3,500, and that it had twelve sections, each of which was an autonomous scientific society, such as the Chinese Dermatology Society, and seven councils, such as the Council on Medical Education. [7]

Up to the time of Liberation, traditional physicians were not accepted as members of the CMA. In 1953, however, reportedly as a result of a directive from Mao Tse-tung, the CMA set up a special liaison committee with traditional doctors, and by 1956 membership in the CMA was opened to them. [8] Unlike the pattern in the Soviet Union, in which separate professional medical associations were abolished after the revolution, [9,10] the CMA remained exclusively a doctors' organization. Other professionals maintained their own societies; for example, the *Chinese Medical Journal* in July 1964 reported the annual meeting of the Peking branch of the Nurses' Association of China.[11]

In the 1960s the journal described the activities of the CMA and the work of its committees, such as the Committee on Exchange of Experience between Traditional Chinese and Modern Medicine, which discussed the establishment of a national association of traditional Chinese medicine and the publication of an official journal,[12] and the Committee for Popularization of Medical Science, which organized a medical team to give lectures on measles, ascariasis, and other medical topics "to medical workers and peasants in the communes," and "to provide consultations."[13]

Canadian physicians visiting China in 1965, just before the start of the Cultural Revolution, found the CMA to be

> . . . an entirely independent self-regulating organization. The total membership is 20,000, and the rough estimate given to us was that there are a million and a half doctors in China. Qualified doctors do not automatically belong to the CMA. Membership is sponsored and there are criteria for qualifications. Enrollment usually stems from the six-year trained physicians. The main tasks of the CMA are: (a) publication of medical journals; (b) arrangements for domestic medical conferences; and (c) organization of international exchanges of medical personnel and information. There is a tenuous arrangement with government whereby they may call on government for financial assistance to promote the CMA's activities, including building and library funds. Traditional medical practitioners can join the CMA but they also have parallel organizations of their own.[14]

The Canadian visitors also described a "Union of Chinese Medical Workers," composed of physicians who had completed a four-year, Western-type training program. This union, the visitors were told, had a membership of several hundred thousand. The union was not mentioned to us during our visits and it is not clear what its current activities are, or whether it still exists.

Some but not all of the changes brought about by the Cultural Revolution were foreshadowed in the summary of the March 1963 meeting of the General Committee of the CMA, which "endorsed the work of the association during the past seven years and discussed its future tasks." These tasks included strengthening the rural *and* the academic work of the CMA, increasing the "popularization of medical knowledge," and continuing "to raise the level of class consciousness by studying the policies of the party and the works of Mao Tse-tung." [15]

Since the Cultural Revolution the CMA, along with all major institutions, has been going through a period of reexamination and modification of its purpose and structure. For example, qualifications for membership are being reexamined. Formerly, we were told, the qualifications were "elitist" and many physicians who wished to join were not accepted. The question of a single association for all health workers is also now under review. Another change, we were told, was that in the past the CMA was supported largely by membership dues; now it receives substantial funds from the government.

As another consequence of the Cultural Revolution, the publications of the CMA were altered markedly, as it was charged that scientific publications were used for the "fame and gain" of the authors rather than for the dissemination of information. Publication of its specialty journals was curtailed, and in October 1966 *China's Medicine* displaced the *Chinese Medical Journal*. The new journal, which ceased publication at the end of 1968, included material such as:

—The works of Chairman Mao Tse-tung, the greatest Marxist-Leninist of our era, who had led the Chinese people's revolution from victory to victory.

—Experience in medical research and clinical practice guided by the invincible thought of Mao Tse-tung.

—Reports on implementation of the policy of medicine in the service of the workers, peasants, and soldiers; prevention first, and health work in integration with mass movements, especially the prevention and treatment of commonly seen diseases in the countryside.

—Advances in the synthesis of modern medicine and traditional Chinese medicine.

—Experience in the Patriotic Health Movement on the part of the masses of the people.

—New people and new things on the medical front resulting

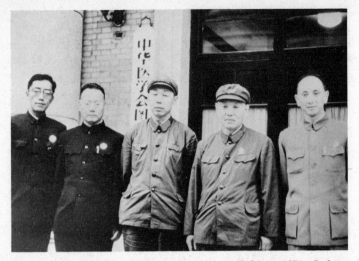

Headquarters, Chinese Medical Association, Peking, 1971. Left to right: Dr. Hsu Chia-yu, interpreter and internist from Shanghai; Kao Chin-o, cadre, CMA; Ma Ching-feng, member responsible for professional work; Hsieh Hua, responsible member, revolutionary committee; and Hsu Shou-jen, secretary-general.

from the creative study and application of Mao Tse-tung's thought.[16]

In 1971 the CMA was led by a revolutionary committee of the usual three-in-one combination: members of the PLA, cadres, and the mass—in this instance, doctors. It was run by a collective leadership, we were told, and all major issues were discussed thoroughly in committee. In 1972, in addition to Hsieh Hua and Hsu Shou-jen of the Ministry of Health, the leadership of the CMA included Fu I-ch'eng, a deputy secretary-general of the CMA, who was deputy leader of the CMA delegation to the United States in October 1972.

In January 1973, with the resumption of publication of the *Chinese Medical Journal* under the auspices of the CMA, the association appears to be assuming its former role as a major vehicle for postgraduate education and the communication of new information to physicians in China and elsewhere. The CMA has a branch in each province, autonomous region, and centrally administered city (see Table 2, page 42); these chapters sponsor regular local meetings, and their representatives meet periodically to compare and coordinate their units' activities. The future role of the specialty groups, which played an important role in the CMA prior to the Cultural Revolution, is not clear, but it may be significant that Dr. Wu Wei-jan, the leader of the 1972 CMA delegation to the United States, was identified as vice-chairman of the Society of Surgery of the CMA.

RESEARCH

Most research in China is directed and supported through the Chinese Academy of Sciences (Academia Sinica), which sponsors a number of institutes, including the Biochemical Institute in Shanghai which startled the world with its total synthesis of biologically active insulin, the Plant Physiological Institute in Shanghai, and the botanical and microbiological institutes in Peking.[17]

Leadership in medical research is the responsibility of the Chinese Academy of Medical Sciences (CAMS), which is directly under the jurisdiction of the Ministry of Public Health. In agricultural research, in analogous fashion, leadership rests with the Chinese Academy of Agricultural Sciences under the Ministry of Agriculture. While both of these academies are administratively separate from the Academy of Sciences, they do work closely with it.[18] The institutes under the jurisdiction of CAMS in 1961, and the list given us in 1972, are tabulated in Appendix K.

In Peking, CAMS sponsors the four research and teaching hospitals described in Chapter II, including the Capital Hospital. The library of the academy is located in one wing of that hospital, in one of the buildings of the former Peking Union Medical College. The library appears extremely extensive and up-to-date, with current issues of major medical journals from all over the world. Among the leaders of CAMS with whom we talked was Wu

Chieh-ping, a urologist at the Capital Hospital and deputy chief of the academy.

In Peking we also visited the Institute of Materia Medica, which is now concerned mainly with extraction and analysis of active principles of traditional medicines. The institute's work is described in the next section. During the Cultural Revolution a number of staff members of the institute had gone to work in rural areas, but by the time of our 1971 visit the institute appeared to be resuming its full activities. Researchers told us that almost all research is now "mission-oriented," but that a sound idea can usually get support if it is related to one of the areas felt to be of high priority.

Medical research is also carried on in the medical schools. In addition to the research on traditional medicine that we observed in every medical school we visited, other areas of intensive research interest are the "common illnesses," including bronchitis and cancer. Departments of public health in the medical schools conduct research on health care needs, on new methods of health care delivery, and on occupational illnesses.

The research being conducted at the Sian Medical College in 1972 seems typical of that currently being conducted in medical schools in China. The professor of physiology, Hou Chung-lin, showed us, for example, neurophysiological experiments on rabbits in order to determine the method of conduction of acupuncture stimulation. A point in the rabbit's paw, comparable to the *hoku* point in man, was needled, and the resulting impulses measured in the ulnar nerve, using advanced electronic amplification and oscillographic equipment.

Another example of the work in progress at Sian was shown us in the Department of Pharmacology, where research was being conducted to develop better methods for treating chronic bronchitis, based on traditional herb medicines. The Department of Chemistry at the college had made extracts from herbs which were used empirically to treat bronchitis. These medicines were then tested on mice into whose peritoneal cavities a blue dye had been injected. The amount of blue dye obtained in washings of the bronchial tree was used as a measure of the effectiveness of the extracts in reducing bronchial secretions.

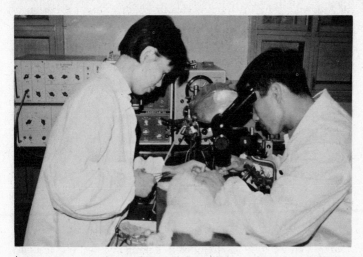

Acupuncture experiments being performed on a rabbit at Sian Medical College.

An area currently emphasized in research is that of occupational health. Research institutes and medical colleges work closely with the city or provincial organizations responsible for occupational safety, as well as with the factories concerned. In a study of the health hazards of argon-arc welding, for example, the Institute of Health of CAMS collaborated with the Peking Anti-Epidemic Health Station, which, despite the implications of its name, also has responsibility for the prevention of noninfectious disease, and with the Peking Metal Structure Factory. Their work included measurement of the ozone concentration in air breathed by the welders, determination of the amount of high-frequency electromagnetic radiation to which the workers are exposed, physical examination of long-time welders, experiments with animals breathing comparable concentrations of ozone, and the testing of various protective devices. The results of their studies and their recommendation for a maximum allowable concentration of ozone—which they showed can be achieved with specific protective measures—were published in the *Chinese Medi-*

cal Journal.[19] The Institute of Health of CAMS has a Division of Occupational Health, which recently reported on the use of a fibrous filtering membrane for sampling dust concentration produced in rock drilling,[20] and a Division of Environmental Health, which recently reported on pollutant gases emitted from diesel engines.[21]

An Institute of Traditional Chinese Medicine was listed as being under the jurisdiction of CAMS in 1961. An example of the work of the institute is the treatment of cataracts by "modified traditional cataractopiesis," as reported in 1968.[22] In 1971 we were told that while there is an institute with that name, it is not part of CAMS. The institute was said to be "on the same level" as CAMS, both being under the jurisdiction of the Ministry of Health. Our informants were probably referring to the Academy of Traditional Chinese Medicine, which, according to two members of its Department of Medical History writing in *China Reconstructs* in July 1973,[23] was founded in Peking in 1955. The academy now has two research institutes—traditional pharmacology and acupuncture—three hospitals, and a medical school. The authors state that "research institutes of traditional Chinese medicine had been set up in most provinces and municipalities."

An article in the March 1973 issue of the *Chinese Medical Journal,* credited to the "Antidiphtheria Mixture Research Group, Institute of Chinese Materia Medica, Academy of Traditional Chinese Medicine, Peking," discusses the production, standardization, and storage of a traditional mixture said to have "practically the same efficacy as diphtheria antitoxin in localized pharyngeal diphtheria." [24] The May 1973 issue of the same journal cites the Kuang An Men Hospital "of the Academy of Traditional Chinese Medicine, Peking" and the urology department of the Peking Friendship Hospital as the sources of an article on the treatment of tuberculous cystospasm by combined traditional and Western methods.[25]

The results of the Cultural Revolution's attack on the publication of articles serving individual "fame and gain" are evident in the new *Chinese Medical Journal.* Of the forty-six major articles in the first four issues (January to April 1973), only five are credited to individual authors; all the others give as their sources simply the name of a research group, laboratory, or department of a hospital, medical college, or research institute. These range from the "Department of Surgery, Workers' Hospital of the Meishan Construction Site, Meishan," which reports on the successful treatment of a single patient with an extensive, deep burn,[26] to the "Department of Surgery, Tumor Institute of the Chinese Academy of Medical Sciences, Peking," which reports on a study of the treatment of 1,230 patients with cancer of the esophagus and stomach.[27]

PHARMACEUTICAL RESEARCH AND MANUFACTURING

Major research efforts are being devoted to the practical purpose of finding the most effective drugs for common diseases. At the Institute of Materia Medica, over 300 workers are doing basic research on drugs for such illnesses as the common cold, bronchitis, hypertension, cardiovascular disease, and cancer. The institute has departments of pharmaceuticals (chemical synthesis), phytochemistry, pharmacological research, pharmacological analysis, and medicinal plants. Research workers are exploring the "treasurehouse" of traditional Chinese medicine, collecting herbal remedies, and subjecting them to analysis to determine their active ingredients. Among the drugs being investigated are herb medicines for poliomyelitis and Bell's palsy, cardiac drugs, reserpine and other drugs for hypertension, antitumor drugs, and oral contraceptives.

The researchers perform clinical trials of the drugs on hospitalized patients, we were told, only after thorough investigation and self-experimentation, and with the explicit permission of the patient. They also oversee the production of drugs in factories, and return regularly to the hospitals to observe their effects on patients. Thus there is an attempt to tie research closely to the implementation of its results.

Before the Cultural Revolution, we were told, the institute did research only; now it also trains researchers. Our hosts stressed that there is less distinction than in the past between the status of technical and professional personnel. We were given the impression of "scientists" and "technicians" working side-by-side.

Before Liberation only a few drugs were manufactured or processed in China; most pharmaceuticals, except for herb medicines, were imported and expensive. The Chinese pharmaceutical industry has developed rapidly since Liberation, and a fairly comprehensive system has evolved for carrying on scientific research, designing factory construction and technological processes, manufacturing the needed equipment, and producing drugs. The number and variety of drugs have increased immensely and prices have been reduced repeatedly. It is reported that China is now producing all the major materials it needs for the prevention and treatment of disease, and to be exporting medicines to other countries. It is now basically self-sufficient in the chemicals needed for pharmaceutical production. Special efforts have been made by the industry in the last few years to produce drugs for distribution in the rural areas. The production of drugs from traditional medicinal herbs, as well as Western medications, has increased rapidly. In 1971 the national output of sulfanamides, antibiotics, antipyretics, antituberculosis drugs, hormones, and vitamins, was reported to be more than double that of 1966 when the Cultural Revolution started.[28]

During our visit to the Peking Institute for Biological Products—located about fifteen miles outside the city—we were shown some the the modern production facilities. We were told that the institute, which employees 600 people, produces "vaccines" against pertussis, diphtheria, tetanus, smallpox, poliomyelitis, measles, influenza, brucellosis, Japanese B encephalitis, and meningococcal meningitis Groups A and B (see Chapter II). While yellow fever vaccine is also produced, it was carefully pointed out to us that it is manufactured only for export to Africa since there is no yellow fever in China. The institute also produces diagnostic sera, including a simple, rapid, inexpensive, effective test for the diagnosis of pregnancy from a single drop of urine.

The institute serves the needs of the cities of Peking and Tientsin, the provinces of Hopei (in which Peking and Tientsin are located) and Shansi (west of Hopei), and the Inner Mongolian autonomous region (northwest of Hopei). We were told that six additional facilities, similar in size and organization to the Peking institute, serve the rest of the country.

In the past few years unified drug prices have been set throughout China, and in 1969 the price of drugs was reduced by 37 per cent. Medicines are said to be one-fifth of their cost in the early 1950s. Vaccines, drugs for children, and oral contraceptives are supplied free of charge.[29]

NOTES

1. Tillman Durdin, "China Again Fills Cabinet Post from the Ranks of the Military" *New York Times* (December 31, 1972).

2. *Xinhua* (New China) News Agency, "Shanghai Improves Environment," (September 27, 1972).

3. Durdin, "China Again Fills Cabinet Post."

4. "China Takes Part in World Health Assembly," *Ta Kung Pao* no. 364 (May 10-16, 1973): 2.

5. "Peking Names Woman as Minister of Health," *New York Times* (June 21, 1973): p. 4.

6. "The Chinese Medical Association," *Chinese Medical Journal* 46 (1932): 86-88.

7. Szeming Sze, *China's Health Problems* (Washington, D.C.: Chinese Medical Association, 1943): p. 50.

8. Ralph C. Croizier, *Traditional Medicine in Modern China* (Cambridge: Harvard University Press, 1968): p. 177.

9. Mark G. Field, *Soviet Socialized Medicine* (New York: Free Press, 1967): p. 58.

10. ——— "Taming a Profession: Early Phases of Soviet Socialized Medicine," *Bulletin of the New York Academy of Medicine* 48 (1972): 83-92.

11. "News and Notes: Annual Meeting of Peking Nurses' Association," *Chinese Medical Journal* 83 (1964): 481.

12. "News and Notes: Exchange of Experience between Traditional Chinese and Modern Medicine," *Chinese Medical Journal* 83 (1964): 409.

13. "News and Notes: Popularization of Medical Knowledge," *Chinese Medical Journal* 82 (1963): 400.

14. David M. Baltzan and W. Stuart Maddin, "Medicine in China," *Canadian Medical Association Journal* 93 (1965): 1118-22.

15. "News and Notes: Meeting of the CMA General Committee," *Chinese Medical Journal* 82 (1963): 260.

16. "To Our Readers," *China's Medicine* no. 1 (January 1967): 74.

17. Ethan Signer and Arthur W. Galston, "Education and Science in China," *Science* 175 (1972): 15-23.

18. Leo A. Orleans, "Research and Development in Communist China," *Science* 157 (1967): 392-400.

19. Institute of Health of the Chinese Academy of Medical Sciences, Peking Anti-Epidemic Health Station and Peking Metal Structure Factory, Peking, "Studies on Health Hazards in Argon-Arc Welding," *Chinese Medical Journal* no. 3 (March 1973): 40.

20. Division of Occupational Health, Institute of Health, Chinese Academy of Medical Sciences, Peking, "The Use of Fibrous Filtering Membrane for Sampling

Dust Concentration and Estimating Dust Dispersion," *Chinese Medical Journal* no. 1 (January 1973): 12.

21. Division of Environmental Health, Institute of Health, Chinese Academy of Medical Sciences, Peking, "A Quantitative Study of Major Pollutants Emitted From Diesel Engines," *Chinese Medical Journal* no. 1 (January 1973): 13.

22. Department of Ophthalmology, Institute of Traditional Chinese Medicine, Peking, "Integration of Traditional Chinese and Modern Medicine to Serve the Health of the Working People," *China's Medicine* no. 2 (February 1968): 107-24.

23. Li Ching-Wei and Tsai Ching-feng, "Traditional Chinese and Western Medicine—from Opposition to Integration," *China Reconstructs* 22, no. 7 (July 1973): 2-5.

24. Antidiphtheria Mixture Research Group, Institute of Chinese Materia Medica, Academy of Traditional Chinese Medicine, Peking, "Pharmaceutical Studies of a Traditional Antidiphtheria Mixture," *Chinese Medical Journal* no. 3 (March 1973): 39.

25. Department of Urology, Peking Friendship Hospital, and Kuang An Men Hospital of the Academy of Traditional Chinese Medicine, Peking, "Combined Traditional and Western Medicine in Treatment of Tuberculous Cystospasm: Report of 4 Cases," *Chinese Medical Journal* no. 5 (May 1973): 65.

26. Department of Surgery, Workers' Hospital of Meishan Construction Site, Meishan, "Successful Treatment of Extensive Deep Burns: Report of a Case," *Chinese Medical Journal* no. 4 (April 1973): 44.

27. Department of Surgery, Tumor Institute of the Chinese Academy of Medical Sciences, Peking, "Study of 1,230 Surgical Cases of Carcinoma of Esophagus and Gastric Cardia," *Chinese Medical Journal* no. 2 (February 1973): 28.

28. "Big Advances in Pharmaceutical Industry," *Peking Review* 15, no. 11 (March 17, 1972): 22.

29. Ibid.

IX. Summary

ALTHOUGH there is still a considerable dearth of information, and probably some misinformation, about China's present health care system and its impact, there can be no doubt that since Liberation the Chinese have made startling progress in the provision of medical care. Severely hampered by lack of resources, manpower, and facilities, the People's Republic of China has placed a high priority on making health care available to its people and, within that objective, the highest priority on preventive medicine and on the delivery of medical care to those who had previously had the greatest difficulty obtaining access to health services. The methods used seem extremely well-suited to the health problems of today's China, and, even more important, they are remarkably well-integrated with the social structure the Chinese are attempting to build. They are recruiting, training, motivating, and employing medical personnel in ways very different from those in the West. Human power is often substituted for technology, but within that context medical personnel appear to be used to their fullest potential. Medical care is considered not only in terms of individual well-being, but in relation to the society and its overall development.

More precise generalizations about current health services are difficult because most services are decentralized—which is itself a very important generalization—and differ markedly from place to place within China. Nonetheless it seems important to attempt to state some specific summarizing principles derived from our observations.

The major question being asked in China, particularly since the Cultural Revolution, is "for whom?"

Although much progress was made from the time of Liberation through 1965, one of the major contentions of the Cultural Revolution was that services—including medicine—were still disproportionately serving the well-educated, the managers, and the urban dwellers, and were in many ways self-serving to the providers of the services. What appeared to some as an attempt to improve the "quality" of services appeared to others as a further diversion of limited resources from the care of those who were relatively poorly served. As a result of the Cultural Revolution a great effort is being made to redistribute current resources, to build new facilities, and to train new personnel so that those who are the least advantaged in the society have the greatest proportionate share. Whether this will reduce, or retard, progress in the "quality" of technological medical care is not certain, but that possibility certainly exists. That the current emphasis will provide better "quality" in the sense of wider availability of care seems beyond doubt.

Great stress is given to the provision of health care in rural areas

Because the rural areas in which 80 per cent of the Chinese people live have been the least served, Mao's 1965 directive, "In health and medical work, put the stress on the rural areas," has become a watchword. As part of their attempt to equalize the quality of life in the cities and in the countryside the Chinese are building great numbers of medical facilities in the rural areas, training large numbers of indigenous health workers, and rotating physicians, nurses, and other personnel from the cities into the countryside. There is still, however, a relative, and frequently absolute, shortage of medical resources in these areas. For example, the ratio of regularly trained doctors to population for China as a whole is still about 1:5,000, a very low ratio compared to that of the technologically highly developed countries. Since the major municipalities such as Peking and Shanghai have ratios close to 1:1,000, the ratio in the rural areas is probably even lower than that for the entire country. Nonetheless, substantial increases in the number of health workers have been accomplished in China as a whole over the past two decades, and in the rural areas over the past few years.

Each commune is still expected to be relatively self-sufficient with regard to its health services, but its resources are markedly strengthened by the assignment of urban physicians and other health workers to the rural areas. The salaries of these workers continue to be paid by their urban units, thus ensuring no loss in income. This technique of transferring manpower rather than money from urban to rural areas avoids some of the implications of dependence, and some of the difficulties rural areas would have in recruiting doctors, even if they had the money to do so. The Chinese apparently have had considerable success in approaching the urban-rural distribution problem, a problem that remains unsolved, not only in poor countries and countries such as the United States, but even in the Soviet Union, which theoretically has the power to assign its vast number of doctors to areas where they are most needed.

Most services and training programs are being decentralized

The Chinese are alleged to have been the inventors of bureaucracy—one of the lesser of the many discoveries the world owes them. The increasing centralization and bureaucracy and the growing distance of managers from the people they serve was another central issue of the Cultural Revolution. Since 1966, medical care services and training facilities for medical personnel have been more and more decentralized to the cities or provinces, and within them to the urban district or rural commune. Within certain broad guidelines each city, province, district, or commune appears to be able to make its own decisions about the nature of the training of health personnel and the ways they are used.

Decentralization is related to an emphasis on local "self-reliance"

The Chinese characters usually translated as "self-reliance" are *tzu-li keng-sheng*—more accurately translated as "regeneration through one's own efforts." Health services, and indeed all human services, are provided at the most local level at which they can possibly be given. What we in the West might call social or welfare services—the care for a disabled older person or for the children of an ill mother—are provided at the family or group level. Primary medical care is given at the residents' committee or lane level by Red Medical Workers. Each person, each family, each courtyard, each village is expected to do as much as it can for itself —and to be transformed and strengthened by the process.

Strong referral pathways and specific lines of authority and responsibility are maintained

The decentralized health services function as well as they do, in our view, because they are part of a highly organized pattern that provides specific lines of authority and responsibility, and clear pathways of referral of patients to sources of secondary care and then back to sites of primary care. There appears to be a reasonable amount of supervision of the work of locally based facilities, and opportunity for local workers to receive advice and continuing education from more specialized personnel. Conversely, there are clear channels through which higher levels of organization receive reports and criticism from local levels.

Central policy direction is clearly present, but its post-Cultural Revolution structure is not yet clear

From conversations in China and inferences from other materials and observations—but not yet from formal published documents—it appears that the national Ministry of Health, and its provincial and municipal counterparts, are nearing the end of their process of post-Cultural Revolution transformation and are again playing an important role in gathering data and setting overall policy in the health field. Much, however, that we in the United States would view as policies to be set at a national level—such as educational standards for specialty training—are still determined on a local level. Despite great variation in practices, however, the principles expressed, particularly those quoted from Chairman Mao, vary little from one area to another.

Major efforts are being made to integrate traditional Chinese medicine with Western medicine

Although attempts were made from the time of Liberation to bring together traditional Chinese medicine and "modern" Western medicine, relatively little had been accomplished up to 1966. Since the start of the Cultural Revolution the two types of medicine have been increasingly integrated, both in practice and in education. Under the impetus of Mao's instructions to "make the past serve the present and foreign things serve China," and to "weed through the old to bring forth the new," Western-type doctors are being trained in the use of techniques such as acupuncture and in the use of herb medicine, and traditional practitioners are being brought into closer relationship with Western-type institutions and doctors. Although acupuncture, and particularly acupuncture anesthesia, has captured the lion's share of attention in the United States, developments in other areas, such as combined techniques used in the treatment of fractures, and the use of herb medicines for a wide variety of symptoms, may be of even greater significance. While the "quality" of some of the traditional Chinese medical practices has been criticized in China, and while the absence of controlled clinical trials has been deplored by Western observers, it seems likely that the active exploration and wide use of traditional methods will not only continue but very likely lead to new insights into the treatment of illnesses.

Prevention of illness is stressed, and is closely tied to medical care

The same facilities that provide medical care locally—the lane stations in the cities, the production brigade stations on the communes, and the stations in the factories—have responsibility for preventive services. Likewise, the duties of the health workers who provide medical care—the doctors, nurses, barefoot doctors, worker doctors, Red Medical Workers, and health workers—also include preventive services. Thus the opportunities provided in the delivery of personal medical care are used to promote preventive medicine, and vice versa. The multilevel, geographically based structure of the system leads to medical

personnel being responsible for communities rather than only
individual patients, and the fact that they are salaried means
they are not dependent on fee-for-service payments for individual,
curative, or ameliorative medical care as motivation for their
efforts. There still appears to be much work to be done in control
of preventable infectious diseases such as trachoma, tuberculosis,
and parasitic infestations, as well as in the prevention of degenerative diseases, such as cancer and stroke, that appear to be replacing
infectious diseases as the major causes of death.

The mass is mobilized to participate in their own health care and that of their community

The Chinese make extensive use of essentially untrained
community members in health and medical care. These individuals, who are called mass workers, volunteers, nonprofessionals, or spare-time workers, depending on the context, participate in the "great patriotic health movements" and are
expected to play a leading role in carrying out public health
measures as well as in their own medical care. Other examples
are the rural health workers trained by barefoot doctors, who
do environmental sanitation and other work during their lunch
breaks and leisure time. Great stress is also placed on health
education, on individual responsibility in prevention of illness,
on overcoming one's illness when sick, and on caring for one's
neighbors when necessary.

A broad spectrum of medical care personnel is being developed

The purpose of attempting to develop and use every individual to the highest level of his capacity is not only to achieve
maximum use of human potential in a people-rich, technology-
poor society, but the fulfillment of the ideological goal of providing opportunities for each person to "serve the public first, self
second." The object is not only to provide additional manpower
for health services, but to transform the attitudes of those who,
perhaps for the first time in their lives, are given the opportunity for useful, helping roles. One corollary to this philosophy
is the development of a broad spectrum of skills—ranging from

community members with no special training or skills to super-specialists who have a different attitude toward community service than do many of their Western counterparts. Any single health worker can play a number of roles, some very different from our Western models.

Emphasis is placed on skills rather than on credentials

Another corollary to the use of each individual to his fullest capacity is that the skills a person demonstrates seem considerably more important than the length of his training, his experience, or the possession of a specific license or credential. Thus we saw health workers trained as doctors, assistant doctors, and nurses all doing comparable work in ambulatory care settings, often working side-by-side.

The decentralized nature of education and employment would make nationwide standards for either very difficult to achieve, even if that were one of the Chinese goals. Since role assignment and promotion are usually on a local level, it seems quite possible that these decisions can be made on the basis of direct observation and evaluation of the skills of the person involved. The use of barefoot doctors in the communes, worker doctors in the factories, and Red Medical Workers in the neighborhoods—all of whom play dual roles—is consistent with the principles of training personnel just up to the level needed for the performance of specific tasks, of emphasizing prevention rather than treatment, and of attempting to minimize the barriers caused by educational and status differences between health workers and the people they serve.

Whether these patterns will continue as technology develops and as expectations of technical expertise increase is unclear. In 1972 some people in the cities were already criticizing the "poor standards" and "mistakes" of the barefoot doctors, and evidencing concern over how they might be improved. But for the present there are said to be over a million barefoot doctors, and peasants are "quoted" as saying of them: "With medicine packs on their backs, they are our trusted doctors; with hoes on their shoulders, our good commune members; and when coming home, our heart-to-heart families." [1] They are not likely to be displaced or replaced very easily, even if the Ministry of Health or other authorities should want to do so.

There have been major changes in the recruitment and training of doctors of Western medicine

Faced with a very inadequate supply of doctors, after Liberation the Chinese began to train a large number of doctors following Western and, especially, Soviet patterns, a policy that was harshly criticized during the Cultural Revolution. Since the Cultural Revolution the duration of medical training has been reduced from the previous six or eight years to three years or less, and the curriculum has been drastically altered. This has been accomplished by removing from the curriculum the "irrelevant" and the "redundant" and by using new methods of teaching that require the active participation of the students. The method of recruitment into medical school has also undergone changes: Candidates are selected by their fellow workers in the communes and factories, and barefoot doctors and other health workers are being given increased opportunities for medical school training.

In medical education, too, in 1972 we observed some shift away from the situation as it had been in the previous year. Many more medical schools had been reopened by the fall of 1972, and while nominally sticking to a "three-year" program, as had been urged by Mao in 1965, almost all have added a six-month "premedical" course in basic sciences and languages to help make up for the students' inadequate secondary school education in these subjects. Medical student selection seems somewhat more flexible, but it still emphasizes selection by peers in communes and factories, with criteria of service and ideological attitude outweighing academic credentials. Previous health work experience as a barefoot doctor or nurse is a common factor of many students.

Education still emphasizes the practical relative to the theoretical, with a major part of the training taking place at the commune or county level where students, supervised by their teachers, work with patients and local health workers. Medical students pay no tuition, receive a modest stipend during training, and are expected to return to their units to work after graduation.

Medical research is predominantly "applied research"

Although research in 1972 showed some return to pre-Cultural Revolution patterns, work on techniques of traditional Chinese medicine, particularly herbs and acupuncture, and on treatment of common illnesses is still being emphasized, and this policy shows little evidence of change. The changes one observes are more subtle, such as the presence on the delegation of Chinese physicians who visited the United States in the fall of 1972 of an Academy of Medical Sciences researcher whose field is the basic biochemistry of cancer, and the emphasis in the *Chinese Medical Journal* on specific technological advances rather than on patterns of care for sick people or for communities. Even so, the highest priority in medical research in China for the foreseeable future will most likely lie in applied research that offers the promise of short-run practical results rather than in "basic research." In general the major effort appears to be in finding ways to extend the availability of that which is already known to as many people as possible; the exploration of the not-yet-known and the not-yet-relevant is given relatively less attention.

Production and distribution of pharmaceutical and other medical supplies has improved markedly and appears to be approaching self-sufficiency in many categories.

In contrast to the pharmaceutical industry in a country such as the United States, with its high costs based on large research and advertising budgets and/or on high profits for the manufacturer, medicines in China are falling rapidly in price and are for the most part extremely inexpensive; in contrast to the industry of a country such as the Soviet Union, with its inefficiencies of production and distribution and periodic shortages, the industry in China appears to be extremely well-organized and productive; in contrast to other technology-poor countries that are dependent on wealthy countries for their supplies, the Chinese appear to be self-sufficient in most important items. Even in the area of development of new products and methods of production, where one might expect the greatest difficulties, China appears to be making rapid progress. To what extent and how this has been accomplished over such a short span of time is not fully understood; it is a little discussed but apparently exciting special area of Chinese accomplishment worth considerable further exploration.

Salary structures have been altered in the wake of the Cultural Revolution

With the exception of the barefoot doctors, who participate in the income and produce distribution system of the communes, all medical personnel in the cities and the rural areas are now on salary—a change from the persistence of some private practice into the early 1960s. Salary and status differences among medical personnel with different levels of expertise are apparently being reduced. Prior to the Cultural Revolution, following the Soviet pattern, great salary differentials had developed. Doctors who were particularly senior in specialization or in academic status often earned four to five times as much as a beginning doctor, and experienced doctors earned considerably more than experienced nurses or other health workers. One result of the Cultural Revolution has been a decision that wages at the upper end of the range will be frozen until wages at the lower end rise to meet them. This is a relatively new policy, and its pattern of application, its consistency, and its effects are not yet clear.

Professionals and intellectuals are being "reeducated"

As part of the effort of the Cultural Revolution to minimize status differences between those who work with their minds and those who work with their hands, all intellectuals spend some periods of time being "reeducated," usually in "May 7th schools" in the countryside. Medical workers, including superspecialists from urban hospitals, spend six months to a year, or longer if they wish to take their families with them, in rural areas, providing services and training other personnel while being themselves educated in all aspects of rural life. From those with whom we talked it seems quite clear that these kinds of experiences have given urban medical specialists a new respect for the problems, the work, and the dedication of the peasants.

There is a strong emphasis on continuing education

The Chinese believe that the formal initial period of training of all medical workers is much less important than continuing on-the-job supervision and training. As an example, the continuing education of the barefoot doctor is considered to be the most important part of his training; whenever possible consultant doctors carefully review with him the care of his patients.

In urban areas, at least, some choice of source of care seems available to patients

Although choice in the rural areas is of course limited, the ambulatory patient in the city seems to have a choice of using his local residents' committee or lane health station, the ambulatory services of the neighborhood or district hospital, the hospital emergency room, and, if he is a worker or a dependent, the medical care facilities of the factory. We were surprised to be told in Peking that there was considerable concern about the "inappropriate" use of emergency rooms by patients seeking medical care for nonurgent conditions, so there is clearly some choice available.

Methods of payment for care vary widely, but cost does not appear to be a barrier to care

Medical care payment methods range from total subsidization by the patient's employer through payment for individual services by the patient. Certain categories of industrial workers have all their medical care paid for by their factories. Families of factory workers are subsidized for only half the cost of services; the balance is paid out-of-pocket. Peasants on many, but not yet all, communes may participate in a "cooperative medical care system." Each family pays an annual premium into the fund for each of its members and the commune supplements this contribution from general funds; thus the entire family is covered for all medical expenses. Experiments with unsubsidized, prepaid medical care systems—with consequent higher premiums—are being conducted in urban neighborhoods. People pay for individual services, although there are ways for their neighborhood committees to ease the burden.

The Chinese hope to see the elimination of all payments at times of illness "when there are sufficient resources to make this possible." It will apparently be done, as is so much else, on a decentralized basis. The cost of individual services, and of prepayment premiums, is extremely low, even as a percentage of a worker's income; the payments are felt by the Chinese to be little or no barrier to access to care.

The continuity between past and present is maintained

It has been part of Mao's special genius to emphasize continuity rather than discontinuity with the past. The organization of medical care is clearly tied to patterns of social organization, which in turn are closely related to familial, village, and neighborhood patterns of the past. Even reports of new advances in technology stress their continuity with past practices. While much that is old has been criticized and changed, elements have been preserved and integrated into the reality of the present and the vision of the future.

In motivation the emphasis is on the opportunity to be of service rather than on personal reward

Everywhere we went we saw the words *Wei renmin fuwu,* "Serve the People." To the Chinese with whom we spoke it seemed not at all an empty cliché. It is apparently intended as the basis for a way of life and for all human services, including health care. While there is no doubt that health workers gain personal satisfaction from their work, we were told that the gratification comes from the opportunity to be of service to patient and community rather than from academic status or financial reward. To what extent this is the Chinese ideal rather than the Chinese reality cannot be completely clear to the foreign visitor, but we were impressed that the Chinese—to a greater extent than in any other society we know of—are truly attempting to make it a reality.

IMPLICATIONS FOR OTHER COUNTRIES

It has been said that the Chinese experience is peculiar to China, not only because of unique cultural and political factors but because of the special health problems China had to face, and that it therefore holds few lessons for technologically poorly developed countries, and even fewer for technologically developed countries such as the United States. This we dispute.

Albeit in a totally different social, cultural, and economic context, the United States finds itself facing many of the same issues that confronted and still confront the Chinese. Although we have made technological strides whose impact, for good or ill, is almost beyond comprehension, and have in the process become the richest nation on earth, large segments of our society have been excluded from the benefits that wealth and technology might have brought to all.

Persisting in the midst of our affluence we see a rapidly rising rate of social illnesses such as venereal disease, and dysfunctional social activities such as drug abuse; we see poverty and its attendant diseases such as tuberculosis, and attendant scourges such as rat bites and lead poisoning. We see inequality of distribution and inequitable barriers to the use of health services, and a rising alienation and dissatisfaction on the part of the recipients of the services. Increasingly the question of "to whom" society's resources should be devoted is being raised. The issues of massive bureaucracy and governmental remoteness go hand-in-hand with local disorganization and duplication of facilities.

Folk and traditional medical practices accepted by many of our citizens are ignored or ridiculed by medical professionals, rather than used together with "scientific" techniques to help those who are ill. Prevention of illness often takes second place to efforts to ameliorate established illness. An emphasis on "credentialism" not only leads to mismatches between personnel and tasks, but helps to prevent a large group of able people from playing the helping roles they want to play. Individuals and whole communities are kept in ignorance or are intimidated by individual physicians and the medical establishment, and are discouraged from becoming involved in their own care. It is difficult if not impossible to recruit doctors and other health workers into many rural areas and many urban areas of poverty.

Doctors for the most part are recruited from the best educated and highest income strata of society, are often elitist in their attitudes, and their incomes may be an order of magnitude greater than those of other health workers. Continuing education is rarely effectively offered or accepted; and competition for economic rewards, academic honors, or personal gratification is the rule rather than the exception. Conversely, the concept of "self-reliance" or "local initiative" recently expounded by the administration in the United States has a hollow ring to people in communities such as the South Bronx in New York or Chicago's South Side when they see the wealth of some of the suburban communities that surround them.

To say that we have some of the same problems China had, and to some extent still has, does not necessarily mean that the measures with which the Chinese are experimenting can be adopted in the same form in the United States. Based on their experiences with missionary efforts, ranging from the Peking Union Medical College to Soviet assistance in the 1950s, the Chinese would be the first to insist that each society must develop solutions to its problems based on its own social, cultural, and economic backgrounds.

Nonetheless we believe we can gain insights into the solution of our problems from studying the Chinese experience. In the short run, there are even some specific techniques we might learn directly from China, such as:

1. Specialized methods of medical care

    (a) Acupuncture for analgesia during surgical procedures and for treatment of specific medical problems;

 (b) Traditional Chinese medicines, particularly the use of medicinal herbs;

 (c) Exercise and massage;

 (d) Treatment of severed limbs and widespread body burns.

2. Training of health workers

 (a) Choice of students from previously relatively untapped strata of society;

 (b) Opportunities for "upgrading" health workers into "higher" medical occupations;

 (c) Emphasis in training on the practical rather than the theoretical, thereby reducing the length of the initial training period;

 (d) Widespread programs of on-the-job and continuing education.

3. Organization of public health and medical care

 (a) Increased emphasis on preventive medicine, particularly for "social illnesses" such as venereal disease and drug addiction, and for degenerative diseases such as lung cancer;

 (b) Decentralization of services to the most basic possible level, with increased accessibility to appropriate treatment for common and minor illnesses;

 (c) Standardized referral patterns for specialized care, so as to make optimal use of expensive and scarce resources;

 (d) Involvement of people in the provision of their own services through community health education and community health work.

Transfer of the first group of techniques will be relatively easy, although there will of course be some opposition from elements within the profession who view any change with alarm; there will of course be cultists who abuse the techniques and give them an unsavory reputation; and there will of course be problems in transferring a technique such as acupuncture, with its millenia-old history in China, to a different cultural and theoretical context. But these ought to be relatively surmountable barriers to the introduction of and appropriate experimentation with the techniques.

Transfer of the second and third groups of techniques will be much more difficult because the structure of the education of health workers and the organization of the delivery of health services is so closely intertwined with patterns of education, of other human services, and of the society in general. It may be possible to attempt isolated experiments within medicine, but in our view the applicability of these techniques will depend much more on the accomplishment of urgently needed changes in the macrocosm of society than on changes in the microcosm of medicine and public health. Even here we may be able to learn something from the way China has redistributed its wealth and reset its goals.

To take just one example relevant to both medicine and Asia, we, the richest country in the world, currently obtain over one-third of our new physicians from other countries. From July 1971 to June 1972 United States medical schools graduated 9,500 physicians, while 7,140 foreign doctors arrived here or changed status from that of exchange visitor to that of immigrant; 5,000 of them came from Asia.[2] Much of the lure of course lies in the higher salaries paid to doctors in the United States. But not only can Asia ill-afford to send us its doctors, we can ill-afford to receive them because this need is but a symptom of deep-rooted problems in our society. Over the long run our inability to meet our need for physicians at a reasonable cost, and, more important, our inability to share our wealth of resources equitably within or with those outside our society, will hurt us who "have" more than it hurts those who "have not."

For countries less technologically developed than ours there may be even more immediate lessons from China: (1) The importance of establishing the primacy of preventive medicine; (2) the importance of making health care relevant and acceptable to the people for whom it is meant, using folk medicine and traditional techniques where appropriate; (3) the importance of involving everyone in the society in their own health care and that of their communities; (4) the importance of making certain that all are reached by the available resources rather than using these resources to improve the quality of care for a few; and, probably most significant, (5) the importance of the concept of service as an end in itself rather than as a means to private gain. Even for technologically poorly developed countries it is probable, however, that these lessons cannot be learned and applied without learning other, broader lessons from China, lessons on the very nature of the goals and governance of society and the distribution of its wealth.

We in the United States would be short-sighted indeed not to learn all we can from a society that has faced the monumental problems China has had; while they have by no means been solved, China has at least organized itself imaginatively to meet them. We can no longer treat as an object of pity or scorn, as a victim for exploitation, or as an object to which to bring our "enlightened" technology, theology, or ideology, the one-fifth of the earth's population with whom we must share—and labor collaboratively to improve—a shrinking and deeply troubled but still potentially salvageable planet. If we work together, share our resources, and learn from each other we shall restore in a new context the traditional friendship between the American and Chinese people and help to improve the quality of life for them, for us, and for all of our neighbors.

NOTES

1. Chen Wen-chieh and Ha Hsien-wen, "Medical and Health Work in New China." (Unpublished talk given by two Chinese physicians during a visit to Canada in November 1971.)

2. "Inflow of Asian Doctors May Be Wave of Future," *Medical World News* 14, 20 (March 9, 1973).

Medical Institutions and People Visited in 1971

KWANGCHOW (CANTON)

Chinese Medical Association, Kwangtung Provincial Branch
Cha Shih-yun, responsible member
Chen Hui-shing, staff member
Li Shui-fang, staff member
Li Yao, interpreter

Chungshan (Dr. Sun Yat-sen) Medical College
Sun Jin-bun, party secretary
Kou Chou-chuan, vice-chairman
Hsu Hua-mo, instructor in community health
Mao Wen-hsui, professor of ophthalmology
Yan Tang, vice-director, Medical Department, Second Teaching Hospital

Kwangchow Municipal School for Deaf Mutes
Comrade Ho, vice-chairman, revolutionary committee

PEKING

Chinese Medical Association
Hsieh Hua, responsible member
Ma Ching-feng, member responsible for professional work
Kao Chin-o, cadre
Hsu Shou-jen, secretary-general; member, revolutionary committee; accompanied us during visit
Chang Ching-lien, staff member
Yin Yu-chow, staff member
Wang Lian-shen, staff member
Kan Hsing-fa, interpreter

Peking Medical College
Chu Chian-gun, professor
Wu Shen-yi, professor of otolaryngology

210

Third Teaching Hospital, Peking Medical College
> Chou Kuan-han, surgeon, chief of Acupuncture Anesthesia Unit
> Wu Chen-i, professor of psychiatry
> Shen Yu-chun, director, Department of Psychiatry

Youyi (Friendship) Hospital
> Chiang Ray-ling, Department of Internal Medicine
> Yang Chia-sung, Department of Internal Medicine

Institute of Materia Medica, Academy of Medical Sciences
> Kao Hsi-jung, chairman, revolutionary committee
> Sung Chin-hin, deputy chairman
> Lei Hai-p'ing, pharmacologist
> Hung Liang, organic chemist

Handicraft Factory
> Liu Chung-sun, worker doctor

Shuang Chiao (Double Bridge) Sino-Cuban Friendship People's Commune
> Liu Jian, responsible member, leading body, commune health center
> Liu Yu-sheng, barefoot doctor
> Chang Gui-rong, barefoot doctor
> Chou Shu-ping, midwife

Other Institutions
District General Hospital, West District
Institute for Biological Products
Other Individuals
> Kuo Mo-jo, vice-chairman, Standing Committee, National People's Congress; president, Chinese Academy of Sciences
> Wu Chieh-ping, deputy chief, Chinese Academy of Medical Sciences; urologist, Fanti (Anti-Imperialist), now Shoutu (Capital), Hospital
> Huang Chia-szu, Department of Surgery, Chinese Academy of Medical Sciences
> Lin Ch'iao-chih, chief, obstetrics and gynecology, Fanti Hospital

Fang Hsin, cardiologist, Fanti Hospital

Wu Teh-cheng, urologist, Fanti Hospital

Wu Ying-kai, cardiac surgeon, Fu Wai Hospital

Hsu Yin-hsi, otolaryngologist, Gong-Nong-Bing (Worker-Peasant-Soldier) Hospital

Li Yuan-teh, ophthalmologist, Gong-Nong-Bing Hospital

Chu Hsien-yi, endocrinologist, former dean, Tientsin Medical College

Ma Hai-teh (George Hatem)

Hans Muller

SHANGHAI

Chinese Medical Association, Shanghai Branch

Hong Ming-gui, responsible member

Chiang Jen-kuan, responsible member

Shanghai Machine Tool Factory

Sing Sing Production Brigade, Ma Chao People's Commune

Ho Shi-cheng, barefoot doctor

Chow Sing, barefoot doctor

Chiang Dao-jin, barefoot doctor

Hu Wen-shio, barefoot doctor

Kao Ning-zhin, midwife

Dongfanghong (East Is Red), now Juichin, Hospital, Shanghai Second Medical College

Lo Teh-shan, responsible member, revolutionary committee

Kwang An-kwan, professor and chief, Department of Internal Medicine

Hsu Chia-yu, deputy chief, Department of Internal Medicine; our interpreter during the visit

Ting Wei-yi, Department of Internal Medicine

Huang Shih-kwang, Department of Traumatology and Orthopedics

Chen Da-zhong, Department of Traditional Medicine

Chu Shu-ou, nurse in charge of outpatient department

Shanghai Mental Hospital
>   Dr. Shu, responsible member, revolutionary committee
>   Dr. Ling, member, revolutionary committee

Other Individuals
>   Young Ming-ting, head, Faculty of Public Health,
>   Shanghai First Medical College

HANGCHOW

Chinese Medical Association, Chekiang Provincial Branch
>   Yang Shiao-sun, responsible member
>   Ma Cheng-shen, deputy chairman
>   Tong Da-ping, secretary

Mai Chia Wu Production Brigade of West Lake People's Commune
>   Mai Jen-chai, barefoot doctor

Xiao Ying Hsian (Little Silvery Lane) Health Station

Medical Institutions and People Visited in 1972

KWANGCHOW (CANTON)
    Chinese Medical Association, Kwangtung Provincial Branch
        Cha Shih-yun, responsible member
        Chen Hui-shing, staff member
        Li Shui-fang, staff member
        Chen Han-dee, interpreter
    Other Individuals
        Hu Mong-xian, Department of Public Health, Chung-shan Medical College

PEKING
    Chinese Medical Association
        Hsieh Hua, responsible member; leading member, Ministry of Health
        Kuo Hsing-kuo, responsible member
        Kao Chin-o, deputy secretary-general
        Hsu Shou-jen, deputy secretary-general
        Fan Kuang, responsible member, Peking branch
        Ho Shu-ding, staff member, Peking branch
        Li Chun-yen, interpreter, accompanied us during visit
    Fengsheng Neighborhood Hospital
        Liu Pei-pung, director
        Chi Li-hua, head, Department of Public Health
        Chen Yu-chen, nurse; member of the leading group
        Yang Lan-ying, administrator
        Wei Chuan-ying, staff member
        Tung Wan-hsing, traditional Chinese doctor, Massage Department
        Yu Chiao-chih, traditional Chinese doctor, Surgery Department
        Yang Yi-chin, Internal Medicine Department
    Fengsheng Neighborhood Committee
        Chu Chuang-yin, vice-chairman

Yang Hsio-hua, Red Medical Worker ⎫ Wu Ting
Chang Cheng-yu, Red Medical Worker ⎬ residents'
                                    ⎭ committee

Niu Shu-fang, Red Medical Worker ⎫ Min Kang
Kung Shu-hsin, Red Medical Worker ⎬ residents'
Wang Pei-sheng, Red Medical Worker ⎭ committee

Fengsheng Neighborhood Insulation Material Factory
Chang Liang, chairman, revolutionary committee
Tung Shih-ping, worker doctor

China-Rumania Friendship People's Commune
Feng Yen-chung, leading member, administrative office
Hou Hsiu-ying, head, education and health group
Li Shih-min, responsible member for health
Yin Huan-feng, member, education and health group
Hsiao Hsiu-yun, barefoot doctor, Taipingchiao Production Brigade
Yin Shih-chie, chairman, commune hospital revolutionary committee
Wang Yang-li, barefoot doctor, commune hospital

Shunyi County Hospital
Wang Chan-hao, chairman, revolutionary committee
Chang Hsi, vice-chairman, revolutionary committee
Hsing Jun, responsible member, Surgery Department
Chen Tung-hsiang, responsible member, Shunyi County Bureau of Public Health

Peking Printing and Dyeing Mill
Chang Chun-pao, leading member, revolutionary committee
Chang Han-hua, leading member for health
Jen Hsau-chin, Department of Maternal and Child Health
Tsao Hua-ying, Department of Internal Medicine

Peking Medical College
Ma Hsia, chairman, revolutionary committee
Wang Eh, vice-chairman, revolutionary committee; head, Faculty of Preclinical Sciences
Wang Chih-chun, professor

Hsiao Chuan-fang, head, Department of Environmental Hygiene

Wu Ping-chyuan, instructor in pathology

Lou Chih-ching, professor of pharmacology

Chou Chung-fu, instructor in physiology

Shen Yu-chun, director, Department of Psychiatry

Wu Chen-i, professor of psychiatry

Tse Chi, chairman, revolutionary committee, Department of Public Health

Sung Kung-hua, staff member, administrative office

Yang Hsiang-fu, staff member, administrative office

Shoutu (Capital) Hospital

Hsieh Hsin-pin, pediatrician; vice-chairman, revolutionary committee

Yang Sze-pin, responsible member, professional group

Chang Fen-lan, staff member, responsible for foreigners

Chang Hsiao-chien, chairman, Department of Medicine

Hsu Lo-tien, vice-director, Department of Surgery

Wu Wei-jan, deputy director, Department of Surgery

Ho Tso-hua, vice-director, Department of Gynecology

Other Individuals

Chang Wei-hsun (Arthur Chang), pediatrician; deputy director, Youyi (Friendship) Hospital; now assistant director-general, World Health Organization

Ho Shu-ching, staff member, Peking Bureau of Public Health; responsible for foreign visitors

Liu Kuei, director, Peking Prevention Station; accompanied us during the visit

Ma Hai-teh (George Hatem)

Hans Muller, Peking Medical College

Wu Chieh-ping, urologist; deputy director, Chinese Academy of Medical Sciences

SHIHKIACHWANG

Chinese Medical Association, Hopei Branch

Fu Ta-wei, leading member

Hsiao Li, Shihkiachwang branch

Norman Bethune International Peace Hospital
>   Wang Yung-kuan, director
>   Li Ren-lan, deputy director
>   Han Hsiu-mian, director, Anesthesia Department

SHANSI
>   *Tachai Production Brigade, Tachai People's Commune, Hsiyang County*
>   >   Chen Yong-gui, Communist Party branch secretary
>   >   Chia Cheng-jang, leading member, Tachai brigade
>   >   Kun Fan-sheng, staff member, Tachai brigade
>   >   Liu Chi, physician, director, brigade hospital
>   *Hsiyang County Hospital*
>   >   Wang Ying-chuan, chairman, revolutionary committee
>   >   Li Jua-lin, vice-chairman, revolutionary committee; head, Surgery Department

SIAN
>   *Chinese Medical Association, Shensi Branch*
>   >   Yin Tang-ho, leading member
>   >   Niu Cheng-hsi, leading member
>   >   Kuo Chung-shiao, staff member
>   >   Yu Wen-pin, staff member
>   *Shuan Wang Production Brigade, Shuan Wang People's Commune, Wei Nan County*
>   >   Liu Shih-chai, chairman, revolutionary committee
>   >   Han Chu-ying, director, commune hospital
>   *Sian Medical College*
>   >   Chang Liu-chung, head, educational revolutionary group
>   >   Lan Yin-hsiang, vice-chairman, educational revolutionary group
>   >   Feng Chin-cheng, vice-chairman, educational revolutionary group
>   >   Kuo Jen-yu, instructor in histology and embryology
>   >   Lu Hsin, instructor in pathologic physiology
>   >   Hou Chung-lin, professor of physiology
>   >   Chen Yu-hua, instructor in public hygiene
>   >   Yen Chung-liu, instructor in public hygiene

Ching Nian Lu City Commune (Neighborhood), Lian Hu District
    Ho Kuei-lan, chairman, residents' committee
    Chang Chieh-sheng, vice-chairman, residents' committee
    Hsu Tsu-lian, Red Medical Worker
    Liu Shu-ming, Red Medical Worker
    Sung Yu-ying, Department of Internal Medicine, commune hospital

YENAN

Chinese Medical Association, Yenan Branch
    Liu Yun, responsible cadre
    An Way, interpreter, regional revolutionary committee
Liu Ling Production Brigade, Liu Ling People's Commune
    Li Hung-fu, vice-chairman, revolutionary committee
    Feng Chih-jung, barefoot doctor
    Chang Yao-lung, barefoot doctor
    Chi Meng-ying, midwife
    Tsao Ai-chin, health worker

SHANGHAI

Chinese Medical Association, Shanghai Branch
    Hong Ming-gui, responsible member
    Chiang Jen-kuan, staff member
    Wu Hsiu-chen, staff member
    Wang Ching-tung, staff member
Bureau of Public Health, Shanghai Municipality
    Wang Shi-mong, chief, Department of Curative Medicine, Pharmacy, Hygiene, and Public Health
    Chiang Lian-yi, member, Department of Curative Medicine, Pharmacy, Hygiene, and Public Health
Shanghai Second Medical College
    Hsu Chia-yu, deputy head, Department of Internal Medicine, Juichin Hospital
    Wang Tchen-yi, associate professor of internal medicine, Juichin Hospital
    Pan Chia-hsiang, Department of Gynecology, Third People's Hospital

Jung Yeh-chih, Department of Internal Medicine, Xinhua Hospital

Po Hui-yung, lecturer in anatomy

Mao Ta-chun, assistant in public health

Chao Ching-ying, staff member, revolutionary committee

Fan Ya-fang, staff member, revolutionary committee

Kung Chiang New Village, Yangpu District

Pan Chang-jung, vice-chairman, revolutionary committee

Shai Wen-pei, responsible member, neighborhood hospital revolutionary committee

Chiu Ai, responsible member, neighborhood hospital revolutionary committee

Tong Sui-hsia, staff member in charge of prevention work, neighborhood hospital

Other Individuals

Young Ming-ting, head, Faculty of Public Health, Shanghai First Medical College

Delegation of the Chinese Medical Association
to the United States, October 1972

Dr. Wu Wei-jan, Chairman of the Delegation
Deputy Chief, Department of Surgery
Capital Hospital, Chinese Academy of Medical Sciences (CAMS)
Peking
   (Dr. Wu, a general surgeon, is also vice-chairman of the So-
   ciety of Surgery of the CMA)

Dr. Fu I-ch'eng, Deputy Chairman of the Delegation
Deputy Secretary-General, Chinese Medical Association (CMA)
Peking
   (Dr. Fu, originally trained as a physician, works as an admin-
   istrator of the CMA)

Dr. Chang Shu-hsun
Tuberculosis Research Institute
Peking
   (Dr. Chang is a doctor of traditional Chinese medicine)

Dr. Chou Kuan-han
Deputy Chief, Department of Surgery
Third Teaching Hospital of the Peking Medical College
Peking
   (Dr. Chou is head of the Acupuncture Anesthesia Research Unit
   at the hospital)

Dr. Chu Chuan-yen
Deputy Chief of Obstetrics
Jih Tan Hospital, CAMS
Peking
   (Dr. Chu conducts clinical research on patients with gynecolog-
   ical tumors at Jih Tan, a tumor hospital)

Dr. Han Jui
Institute of Pharmacology, CAMS
Peking

> (Dr. Han, a pharmacologist, conducts research on antitumor drugs)

Dr. Hsu Chia-yu
Deputy Chief, Department of Internal Medicine
Juichin Hospital, Shanghai Second Medical College
Shanghai

> (Dr. Hsu, who speaks fluent English and served as the English interpreter for the delegation and for us during our 1971 visit, is head of the Radioisotope Laboratory at the hospital)

Dr. Li Yen-shan
Lecturer, Department of Internal Medicine
First Teaching Hospital of the Wuhan Medical College
Wuhan

> (Dr. Li is a cardiologist)

Dr. Lin Ch'iao-chih
Professor and Head, Department of Obstetrics and Gynecology
Capital Hospital, CAMS
Peking

> (Dr. Lin, world-renowned for her work in obstetrics and gynecology, is a vice-president of CAMS and a member of the Standing Committee of the National People's Congress of the PRC)

Dr. Liu Shih-lien
Chinese Academy of Medical Sciences
Peking

> (Dr. Liu, a gynecologist, conducts research in the biochemistry of cancer)

Mr. Lu Tsung-min, Secretary to the Delegation
Chinese Ministry of Foreign Affairs
Peking

Dr. Wang Lien-sheng, French Interpreter for the Delegation
Chinese Medical Association
Peking

Dr. Wu Hsueh-yu
Director, Ear, Nose, Throat and Eye Hospital
Shanghai First Medical College
Shanghai
   (Dr. Wu is an otolaryngologist and administrator)

Notes on Dr. Norman Bethune *

Mark Sidel

One of the most revered heroes of the Chinese people is a doctor, Norman Bethune. Although he was at various times a painter, poet, teacher, inventor, writer, and theorist, Norman Bethune was above all a healer.

His father, Malcolm Bethune, a Canadian who came from a long line of Scottish doctors, teachers, and clergymen, turned to the ministry soon after Janet, Norman's older sister, was born in 1888. After Malcolm was ordained the Bethunes moved to Gravenhurst, Ontario, where Henry Norman Bethune was born on March 4, 1890.

For years the Bethunes—including Norman's young brother Malcolm, born in 1893—traveled through small Canadian towns where Norman's father served as a traveling preacher. Their summers were spent at Gravenhurst. It was here that Norman developed his venturesome spirit and his intention of becoming a surgeon. He even dropped his first name, trying to be more like his grandfather who had been one of Toronto's leading surgeons.

Though traveling much of the time, Norman graduated from high school in Toronto and then attended the University of Toronto. During the next few summers he developed a taste for versatility; he worked as a waiter, fireman, reporter, teacher, and lumberjack. He also began to draw, paint, and sculpt. "On my mother's side," he would say, "I'm an evangelist. On my father's side I have a compulsion to do, to act." [2]

When World War I began in 1914, Bethune enlisted, the

---

* This essay on Dr. Norman Bethune is a revised version of a paper written for a ninth grade history course at Horace Mann School; sources include the excellent biography of Bethune written by Allan and Gordon,[1] the only book-length biography of Bethune in English; material in the Norman Bethune exhibition at the Bethune International Peace Hospital in Shihkiachwang; and conversations with Dr. Ma Hai-teh.

tenth man in Toronto to do so, and left for France as a stretcher-bearer. He was wounded at Ypres by a piece of shrapnel in his thigh and spent six months in English and French hospitals.

Following his recovery Bethune finished medical school in Toronto and then enlisted in the British navy and became a lieutenant-surgeon. Six months before the end of the war he requested a transfer and spent the remainder of the war with the Canadian Flying Corps. At the end of the war he arranged to be decommissioned in London.

He arrived in London with only his meager pay from the Flying Corps, but he was soon living lavishly. His love for art took him around Europe buying objects that he would sell for a huge profit in London to maintain his expensive life style. He finished his internship at the Hospital for Sick Children and the Fever Hospital and went to work at a private clinic.

In the fall of 1923 he went to Edinburgh for the examinations for fellowship in the Royal College of Surgeons; there he met Frances Campbell Penney, whom he married a few months later in London. Frances, at twenty-two was very shy, while Bethune, thirty-four, was outspoken and flamboyant; their backgrounds clashed often. Although they loved each other the marriage was not to work out.

They went from London to Canada and then to Detroit where in late 1924 Bethune opened his first practice. Few patients came to his office, however, and he found that most people were afraid to visit him because they could not afford the fees; in fact the only people who could pay were prostitutes. Nevertheless he tried to offer his services to all who needed them regardless of whether or not they could pay.

After seeing Bethune's surgery at a hospital in Detroit, one of that city's leading practitioners suggested that he send his surgery cases to Bethune, who soon began to see patients with much more money. Bethune began to think about his new life and he realized what had happened: While he had formerly been treating the poor he was now treating the rich, but it was the poor who really needed his care. He liked having money, but he had begun to dislike the process by which he made it. He returned to his former practice, driving himself hard to make up for having neglected "his" patients.

At the age of thirty-six he contracted tuberculosis, an almost incurable disease in those days. He divorced Frances, deciding that she should not have to be tied down to a bedridden man, and, feeling condemned to death, went to Trudeau Sanitorium, a well-known institution for the treatment of tuberculosis.

While at Trudeau, Bethune read a book by Dr. John Alexander, who wrote:

> It is rather extraordinary that we should have been so seriously backward in doing pioneer work in the surgery of pulmonary tuberculosis. It will be a surprise to the majority of American physicians who read this book to realize the steady advance in thoracic surgery and the definite hope offered the hopeless.[3]

Alexander went on to say that an operation known as pneumothorax, the insertion of air into a lung to collapse it, could cure tuberculosis in some patients. This operation was performed successfully on Bethune and he was cured.

Bethune now resolved to become a thoracic surgeon. After further study, in January 1929 he joined the staff of the Royal Victoria Hospital in Montreal as a specialist in pulmonary tuberculosis, working under Edward Archibald, one of the leading thoracic surgeons of the day.

Bethune had found a calling. Not content to treat the rich and profit from such a practice, he wanted to help people. Now he was teaching and practicing new surgical techniques to cure pulmonary tuberculosis. Bethune began to invent and modify surgical instruments, beginning with a rib stripper. His instruments were patented, and Bethune's name became well known in the hospitals and institutions where his instruments and techniques were used.[4–6]

Bethune still loved Frances and wanted her back with him again. After months of correspondence she came to Montreal from Edinburgh and they were remarried. Yet a year later she realized that their marriage could not work: Bethune's work was more important to him than anything else. Frances asked for and received a divorce.

In 1933 Bethune took charge of the thoracic surgery department of a large Detroit hospital for a year and gained invaluable
experience. He was then appointed to head a newly formed
thoracic surgery department at a hospital near Montreal. He wrote
to a friend at that time:

> I was appointed Thoracic Surgeon and Bronchoscopist to the
> Sacre Coeur Hospital in Cartierville; 450 beds, twenty miles from
> Montreal. French-Canadian and Catholic. $1200 a year, one day a
> week, so the strain is less strained. My title is: Chef dans les Ser-
> vices de Chirurgie Pulmonaire et de Bronchoscopie! I am going to
> have a nice big white cap made with "Chef" marked in front.
> Really, I am delighted. . . . I cauterized some adhesions there
> yesterday and the chorus of oh's and ah's from the nuns rose like
> a chant at the high altar." [7]

At his clinic Bethune began doing an enormous number of
operations, until he was doing 300 chest operations and treating
1,000 tubercular patients a year.

He had become dissatisfied with the approach most doctors
took to tuberculosis, however, maintaining that it was a disease
of the body and of the environment. It started, he said, with
hunger, poverty, and sickness, and to cure it one would have to
overcome the evils of society. He stated that tuberculosis should
and could be cured in its early stages.

He began to believe in socialized medicine—medicine for the
people—with doctors going to the people, serving the people.
He tried to expose bad health conditions in Quebec and became
known on the breadlines as "Comrade Beth." In 1935 he went
on a study trip to the Soviet Union where he admired the fact that
tuberculosis treatment was free, because it was the patient's right.

In 1936 he established the Montreal Group for the Security
of the People's Health, where he was joined by over 100 doctors,
dentists, nurses, and social workers. He put his research on the
history of medical care and his ideas on health before this group
and they came up with several far-reaching proposals that included national health insurance, free medical care for the unem-
ployed, and teams of health workers to be sent to neighborhoods.

Bethune was visited in 1936 by a member of the Committee
to Aid Spanish Democracy, a group favoring the Loyalists over the

Franco-led Fascists; the committee wanted him to head a medical unit in Madrid. Bethune thought about this offer for a long time. Although he was forty-six he did not want to be on the sidelines. He wanted to be fighting, and in this case healing.

Bethune arrived in Madrid at the beginning of December 1936, when the Fascists were attacking Madrid from all sides. He realized that doctors were needed everywhere, so he formed a medical unit, consisting of himself, an American, and some Spanish doctors, to go to the battle zones to give blood transfusions to the wounded. Thus the first mobile blood transfusion unit was born. Bethune was amazed at the willingness of the people of Madrid to give blood to help their comrades.

Bethune gave transfusions in and near Madrid until the end of January, but he was aware that many of the wounded who most needed blood were at the front. So at the beginning of February the mobile unit set out for Valencia, which was near some of the heaviest fighting, and operated there for several months.

The Republic won its first victory at Guadalajara in early 1937, but still no arms were being sent to the Loyalists from any country except the Soviet Union; arms for Franco were pouring in from Germany and Italy. To raise money Bethune agreed to go on a speaking tour in North America. He arrived in Montreal in June 1937 for a tour that took him from coast to coast in Canada and the United States.

It was now that Bethune first heard that the Japanese were attacking China, trying to add it to their growing empire. Having raised over $50,000 for Spain, Bethune volunteered to take a medical unit to northern China to work with the guerillas. He joined the Communist Party in Toronto before leaving for China on January 2, 1938.

Bethune landed in Hong Kong and flew to Hankow, the seat of the Nationalist Government, where he promptly set out for the territory near Yenan which Mao Tse-tung and his Eighth Route Army had reached at the end of the Long March, and which they were now defending against the Japanese. Bethune traveled by train as far as he could, and then, pursued by the Japanese, started on the 300-mile westward trip to Yenan as a passenger in a mule cart. During the trip Bethune found that it was indeed the policy of the Eighth Route Army to pay for all goods received from the people and for all possessions that had been destroyed. When the mules were killed by Japanese bombs, for example, Major Lee, Bethune's companion, paid $100 (Mexican) to the owners of the cart for each of the dead animals.

Bethune arrived in Yenan at the end of March and was greeted by a delegation headed by Ma Hai-teh (George Hatem), an American doctor who had come to China a few years earlier and who was now medical adviser to the Eighth Route Army. Yenan was a well-run city with a population of approximately 30,000, the headquarters of the Communists and capital of the military region in northern and western China. Yenan had its own medical school and university, and was in fact a model for other cities expected to be built later.

On the night Bethune arrived he met with Mao Tse-tung and suggested the setting up of a mobile unit, not just to give blood but with the equipment and manpower to establish hospitals, perform surgery, and train doctors and nurses. Mao immediately agreed to this plan. Bethune later wrote in his diary:

> As I sat in the bare room opposite Mao, listening to his calm comments, I thought back to the Long March, to Mao as he and Chu Teh had led the Communists on the great trek from the south. . . . I now know why Mao impresses everyone who meets him the way he does. The man is a giant! He is one of the great men of our world.[8]

Bethune spent three weeks in Yenan waiting for his equipment to arrive from Canada. Richard Brown, a young Canadian missionary doctor, also arrived, having taken a three-month leave of absence from his mission hospital in Hankow.

Bethune and Brown immediately set out on an inspection tour of the hospitals in northern Shensi Province. They found the conditions very bad—there were few doctors, little food, and almost no bandages, drugs, and other equipment. Bethune refused to accept the salary that was ordered to be paid to him, putting it instead into a tobacco fund for his patients.

At the end of June they moved eastward into the military

district of Chin-Cha-Chi. The unit was the only mobile medical corps to care for the 13 million people in the 100,000-square-mile district. The 125,000 to 175,000 Chinese soldiers in the area were surrounded by a much larger Japanese force. They arrived at Chiao Tang Chang, the headquarters of General Nieh Yung-chen in the Wu-Tai Mountains, where they spent three weeks inspecting the three base hospitals at Hopei Tsun, Ho Hsi Tsun, and Sheng Yin Kou, where they performed many operations.

To replace Dr. Brown when his leave of absence expired, a former Chinese magistrate named Tung Yueh-chen was enlisted. He was "short, plump, and good-natured. He had the natural tact of a diplomat. He smiled easily." In a week Bethune was calling him "my other self." [9]

General Nieh soon proposed a plan whereby Bethune would organize a medical system for the Chin-Cha-Chi district. For the most part this would consist of establishing small hospitals in towns and villages he visited with the mobile unit. Bethune accepted this assignment immediately. He wrote to Dr. Ma: "I am honored and proud. My title now is Dr. Norman Bethune, Military Adviser to the Chin-Cha-Chi Military District." Soon after his arrival Bethune had also been given a Chinese name, Pai Chu En, meaning "White Seek Grace," in an attempt to transliterate his name as well as to give his Chinese name some meaning.

Work was immediately started on plans for a model hospital in Sheng Yin Kou, the forerunner of many such hospitals, and a campaign was started to make it a reality. Construction proceeded swiftly, and the first operating theater in Chin-Cha-Chi was soon in existence. Bethune helped make sterilizers and supervised a system of sanitation. A plot of ground outside the hospital was turned into a patients' recreation area, and an annex to a Buddhist temple became a hall for games, meetings, reading, and writing. A "learn while you work" program was instituted, and Bethune gave lectures to the peasants and soldiers in the community on medicine, anatomy, the treatment of wounds, and other related topics.

One of his early challenges was to convince the villagers, even the nurses, that it was not dangerous to give blood. He did this by taking his own blood and giving it to a patient in full view of everyone; he received the same response he had gotten in Madrid— the total eagerness of the community to serve their comrades by donating blood.

In one of the early sessions held by the hospital staff devoted to praise and criticism of each other, the nurses and doctors praised Bethune for his work, his leadership, his skill, and his energy, but they had one criticism: he was *chi hsin*—irascible; he would often criticize harshly or sharply. From then on Bethune tried to be less "irascible."

In September, during a period when he was travelling frequently to the front and performing several operations a day, Bethune was called unexpectedly to General Nieh's headquarters. "I have received reports from *every* village, from *every* front you have been at," General Nieh said. "You don't sleep enough. You don't eat enough. And you seem under the impression that no Japanese bullet or shell can come anywhere near you." [10]

A week later the model hospital was officially opened. In his speech Bethune said, "There is an old saying in the English hospitals . . . A doctor must have the heart of a lion and the hand of a lady. That means he must be bold and courageous, strong, quick, and decisive, yet gentle, kind, and considerate." [11] News of the completion of the model hospital spread through Chin-Cha-Chi and Yenan and it was viewed by those at the Communist headquarters as a major breakthrough in the field of medical services for the wounded. The name of Pai Chu En, the foreign doctor, spread through the villages to the front, raising morale throughout the Eighth Route Army.

New fighting soon broke out in the Wu-Tai Mountains. The night before the mobile unit departed, a medical conference established the policy and slogan of all guerilla medical forces: "Our watchword must be: 'Doctors: Go to the wounded. Don't wait for the wounded to come to you!' "

The mobile unit was a well-packed caravan in which each person and animal fitted exactly. At the head of the unit rode Pai Chu En and Tung Yueh-Chen, followed by two other doctors, a nurse, a cook, two orderlies, and two grooms. The unit carried a portable operating table, surgical instruments, anesthetics, splints, and other necessities.

Several days later, they reached Ho Ki Tsun, a first-aid station for the fifth and sixth regiments, and in the six days they were there they did 105 operations. The unit then turned east to Hopei, stopping at towns to tend the wounded and inspect facilities. In mid-October the unit headed for Hung Tsi-tien, only five-and-one-half miles from the front, where the group held a conference to discuss new medical developments. Over the next ten days they traveled 175 miles, visiting thirteen mountain villages. On their return to Chiao Tang Chang, while the others rested General Nieh informed Bethune of recent developments.

The internal situation was very grave. Military reports showed that the Japanese were strengthening their circle around Chin-Cha-Chi and were preparing to mount a stronger offensive. They had captured Hankow and were trying to split the Communist–Kuomintang alliance by appealing to anti-Communist forces within the Kuomintang with peace proposals. At that point General Nieh was wary of an effort by some Kuomintang forces to bottle up the Communists in the north.

The Eighth Route Army strategy was one of continued guerilla warfare: Harass the Japanese, break their communications, and attack from all sides only if victory seems virtually certain. There would be many wounded who would need Bethune's attention. "Already the knowledge of your presence," said General Nieh, "has in itself done much for the morale of our troops."

Soon the unit set out for Chang Yu, where Bethune helped to establish a school of nursing; he also organized a "practical work week" whereby doctors and nurses together swept floors and bathed patients in order to become accustomed to doing menial work. From Chang Yu, in the beginning of November, they travelled northward through the first blizzard of the cold Shansi winter. They passed through Fu Ping, reaching Ho Chien Tsun, the casualty station of the 359th Brigade, on the evening of November 11.

There they were greeted by a Dr. Fong, and Bethune

characteristically asked to see the infirmaries at once. One patient had had a leg wound set so badly that Bethune had to amputate the leg. When he asked who had set the leg originally, Dr. Fong admitted that he had. Bethune became very angry, asking sarcastically, "Tell me, Dr. Fong, what university did you graduate from?"

The next day Tung told Bethune the story of Dr. Fong, having heard it from him the night before. Fong had been born in a small village and had taught himself to read. He became a nurse and then a doctor only by observation: with no formal training, Fong the illiterate had become Fong the *dai-fu*. Bethune apologized to Dr. Fong, realizing that he had learned something about doctors in China. Such an incident did not happen again.

This story was added to the tales that soon grew into a legend about Bethune. Everywhere he went the legend preceded him. Another story was that of the stone and the wounded: At a base hospital situated in a temple the unit found the bottom of a series of stone steps missing.

"Do you mind jumping?" Bethune asked a nearby attendant.

"Not at all," he replied.

"And the convalescing patients—do they mind jumping?"

The attendant's smile vanished. Together they brought a stone to replace the missing step.

On November 27 the unit again left for the battlefront. Starting in the afternoon of November 29 and continuing for eighteen hours, the doctors performed fifty major operations in the midst of the fighting. By the time the battle was won on December 1, the unit had completed seventy-one operations in forty hours. Out of this battle came a new cry: "Attack! Bethune is with us! Bethune is here to take care of the wounded!"

Pai Chu En's name was also spread throughout Japanese-held areas by propaganda agents hoping to destroy the Japanese troops' morale. On December 8 the unit was back in Yang Chia Chang, having traveled 275 miles and performed 113 operations. Of the seventy-one wounded on whom they had operated only one had died.

During this period, Sheng Yin Kou, the site of the first model hospital, had been attacked by the Japanese and the hospital had been destroyed. What happened there is a story of the courage and strength of the Chinese people. The peasants of the village and the surrounding countryside first took all the patients into their huts to share their food and their *k'angs* (a *k'ang* is a stone stove on top of which is a bed). Then they began to dig into the face of a nearby mountain with picks and shovels and cut a long tunnel through the earth and rock. Still with picks and shovels, they built caves leading from the tunnel into the mountain. When the work was finished several months later over 100 caves had been built inside the mountain. Invisible from the ground, inaccessible by air, only those who *knew* where they were could find the caves. This became the new model hospital.

The unit soon found that its supplies and medicines were running low, and none of the hospitals could spare any of theirs. It was up to Bethune to find some way of getting what was needed from Peking, and he persuaded a Protestant missionary to act as his courier.

When most of the fighting switched from Shansi to mid-Hopei early in 1939, Bethune enlarged the unit to eighteen people, brought in Dr. Fong, and set out for the new front. Their destination was Ho Chien, headquarters of the 120th Division of the Eighth Route Army, which was surrounded by the Japanese; the division was ready to evacuate the town at any time. After inspecting the six base hospitals in mid-Hopei it became clear to Bethune that many more doctors were needed and that a permanent medical school had to be started. In a letter to General Nieh, he wrote that of the 200,000 troops in the region, 2,500 were hospitalized at any given time with only fifty untrained Chinese doctors, five graduate doctors, and Bethune to treat them. He suggested reluctantly that he make a trip to North America, as this was the only way to raise the more than $50,000 that was needed. The final decision was made in mid-September: He would leave next month.

At this point his courier returned from Peking with the medicines, but not before the unit had had to operate on fifteen patients without anesthesia. Bethune postponed the trip to North

America until the beginning of November so that he could inspect more of the hospitals. Then, on October 20, the Japanese suddenly attacked Chin-Cha-Chi with 50,000 men in a very large offensive.

On November 2 the unit came to a small village near Mo Tien Ling (Sky-kissing Peak). While there, during the midst of a battle, with patients waiting for surgery, word came that the Japanese were attacking the village, which had very few if any troops left to defend it. Bethune refused to leave and the unit stayed to operate on the remaining patients, departing from the village ahead of the enemy with just moments to spare.

In his haste to complete the operations, however, Bethune had lacerated his finger. The next morning it was badly swollen and he had a high fever. The infection was incised, but septicemia —a general infection—developed. Instead of resting he insisted that they go on. Fong and Tung refused to allow Bethune to operate, and the unit left the next day carrying him on a stretcher to travel through the mountains to the village of Yellow Stone. Allan and Gordon [11] narrate:

> They brought him out of the hills, over the twisting narrow passes where the enemy feared to set foot, and where the horses no longer led but followed . . .
> "It will be Yellow Stone Village," he [Fong] said, pointing, and they began the descent. . . .
> "Pai Chu En!! Pai Chu En!!"
> At the edge of the village the people chanted his name. . . . But as the brown mare reached the gate, and the caravan entered, the shouts of welcome died on their lips. . . . Then they saw the stretcher coming through the gate, and their faces wrinkled with torment and disbelief. . . .
> A shadow glided through the courtyard. "This is the house where Pai Chu En lies?" a voice whispered.
> "We are a detachment of the People's Guard," the soldier said. . . . "Our whole unit has pledged that when we reach the front we will offer ourselves for any duty as an example to the others—self-sacrifice till death, if necessary. . . .
> Tung began to weep quietly, without shame. "Did you know? —This is the second time he is dying, and there are not enough tears in all China to mourn his second passing. . . ."

Fong rose heavily. "Not in all China," he said. "No, Comrade Tung, not in all the world will there be enough tears. . . ."

That morning, as the men were trooping out of the village for the day's labor in the fields, they saw Tung standing in the doorway of Yu's house. They stopped in the courtyard and inquired after Pai Chu En.

"He is dead," Tung said.

It was twenty minutes after five, November 13, 1939. . .

In the valley of East Shansi they built him a tomb. All about were the Japanese, pressing in with their tanks and planes, but by decree of the Chin-Cha-Chi administration and the Eighth Route Army the valley was set aside as an eternal national shrine.

They built it together—soldiers and artists and laborers. They built it with precious marble, stone, and love.

On the four sides of the tomb are four inscriptions:

The internationalist spirit of Comrade Norman
Bethune is worthy to be learned by all Chinese
Communists and by all the Chinese people

Central Committee of the
Communist Party of China

The scientist and revolutionary of the masses

General Nieh Yung-chen

The most valorous fighter on the front of the emancipation of mankind

General Lu Cheng-tsao

The eternal brillance

Tung Yueh-chian

The original site of Bethune's grave in Hopei Province was overrun and destroyed by the Japanese. A memorial tomb was constructed in Shihkiachwang, not far from the original grave and the military hospital in Shihkiachwang, which has grown into a modern medical center serving both military personnel and civilians, is called the Norman Bethune International Peace Hospital.

To honor Bethune, on December 21, 1939, Mao Tse-tung wrote an essay "In Memory of Norman Bethune." This, together with "Serve the People" and "The Foolish Old Man Who Removed the Mountains," has now become one of the "Three

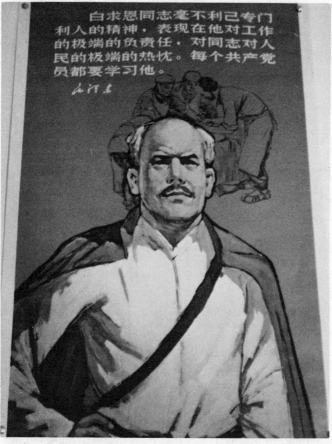

自求恩同志毫不利己专门
利人的精神，表现在他对工作
的极端的负责任，对同志对人
民的极端的热忱。每个共产党
员都要学习他。

毛泽东

Poster in a Peking health station showing Dr. Norman Bethune and
an excerpt from Chairman Mao's essay, "In Memory of Norman
Bethune."

Constantly-Read Articles," which almost all Chinese people read and discuss daily as guides to their work and thought:

> Comrade Norman Bethune, a member of the Communist Party of Canada, was around fifty when he was sent to China by the Communist parties of Canada and the United States; he made light of travelling thousands of miles to help us in our War of Resistance Against Japan. He arrived in Yenan in the spring of last year, went to work in the Wu-Tai Mountains, and to our great sorrow died a martyr at his post. What kind of spirit is this that makes a foreigner selflessly adopt the cause of the Chinese people's liberation as his own? It is the spirit of internationalism, the spirit of communism, from which every Chinese Communist must learn. Leninism teaches that the world revolution can only succeed if the proletariat of the capitalist countries supports the struggle for liberation of the colonial and semi-colonial peoples, and if the proletariat of the colonies and the semi-colonies supports that of the proletariat of the capitalist countries. Comrade Bethune put this Leninist line into practice. We Chinese Communists must also follow this line in our practice. We must unite with the proletariat of all the capitalist countries, with the proletariat of Japan, Britain, the United States, Germany, Italy and all other capitalist countries, before it is possible to overthrow imperialism, to liberate our nation and people, and to liberate the other nations and people of the world. This is our internationalism, the internationalism with which we oppose both narrow nationalism and narrow patriotism.

> Comrade Bethune's spirit, his utter devotion to others without any thought of self, was shown in his boundless sense of responsibility in his work and his boundless warmheartedness towards all comrades and the people. Every Communist must learn from him. There are not a few people who are irresponsible in their work, preferring the light to the heavy, shoving the heavy loads on to others and choosing the easy ones for themselves. At every turn they think of themselves before others. When they make some small contribution, they swell with pride and boast about it for fear that others will not know. They feel no warmth towards comrades and the people but are cold, indifferent, and apathetic. In fact such people are not Communists, or at least cannot be counted as true Communists. No one who returned from the front failed to express admiration for Bethune whenever his name was mentioned, and none remained unmoved by his spirit. In the Shansi-Chahar-Hopei border area, no soldier or civilian was unmoved who had been treated by Dr. Bethune or who had seen

how he worked. Every Communist must learn this true Communist spirit from Comrade Bethune.

Comrade Bethune was a doctor, the art of healing was his profession and he was constantly perfecting his skill, which stood very high in the Eighth Route Army's medical service. His example is an excellent lesson for those people who wish to change their work the moment they see something different and for those who despise technical work as of no consequence or as promising no future.

Comrade Bethune and I met only once. Afterwards he wrote me many letters. But I was busy, and I wrote him only one letter and do not even know if he ever received it. I am deeply grieved over his death. Now we are all commemorating him, which shows how profoundly his spirit inspires everyone. We must all learn the spirit of absolute selflessness from him. With this spirit everyone can be very useful to the people. A man's ability may be great or small, but if he has this spirit, he is already noble-minded and above vulgar interests, a man who is of value to the people.[12]

NOTES

1. Ted Allan and Sydney Gordon, *The Scalpel, The Sword: The Story of Dr. Norman Bethune* (Boston: Little, Brown, and Co., 1952; New York: Liberty Book Club, 1959).

2. Ibid., p. 14.

3. John Alexander, *The Surgery of Pulmonary Tuberculosis* (n.p., 1926).

4. Norman Bethune, "A Plea for Early Compression in Pulmonary Tuberculosis," *Canadian Medical Journal* (July 1932): 36-42.

5. ———, "A Phrenicectomy Necklace," *American Review of Tuberculosis* 26 (September 1932): 319-21.

6. ———, "Some New Thoracic Surgical Instruments," *Canadian Medical Journal* 35 (December 1935): 656-62.

7. Allan and Gordon, *The Scalpel*, p. 60.

8. Ibid., p. 191.

9. Ibid., p. 200.

10. Ibid., p. 213.

11. Ibid., p. 219.

12. Mao Tse-tung, *Five Articles by Chairman Mao Tse-tung* (Peking: Foreign Languages Press, 1968): pp. 5-10.

Analysis of Preliminary Public Health Data for Shanghai, 1972 *

Steven H. Lamm and Victor W. Sidel †

Although changes in a country's birth and death rates and its patterns of demography, morbidity, and mortality are in large measure due to factors other than changes in its health services, statistical changes in these parameters are usually accepted as at least partially due to, and as evidence of, the success or failure of health programs. Statistics from China have in general been neither readily available nor particularly reliable,[1] reflecting, it has been asserted, "a complete indifference to the idea of quantity and a total disregard for any quantitative measurement in Chinese philosophical thinking."[2] While this interpretation is almost certainly overstated, it is indeed true that published statistical data relating to health were meager during the first decade of the People's Republic, and virtually absent during the second. This dearth of official statistical data, particularly since the beginning of the Cultural Revolution in 1966, has led to considerable

* Prepared as a chapter in *China Medicine As We Saw It,* a publication of the Geographic Health Studies Branch, John E. Fogarty International Center for Advanced Study in the Health Sciences, National Institutes of Health, U.S. Public Health Service, U.S. Department of Health, Education, and Welfare, forthcoming.

The authors are grateful for the assistance of: Robert J. Armstrong, chief, Mortality Statistics Branch, Division of Vital Statistics, National Center for Health Statistics, for his aid in calculating the life table for Shanghai; Robert L. Heuser, chief, Natality Statistics Branch of the division, for his help in intepreting the data on plural births; Edward B. Perrin, deputy director of the center, and Robert A. Israel, director of the division, for their advice on the handling of the data and their encouragement in the preparation of this report; Haitung King, Morton Schweitzer, and Carl W. Tyler for their comments on the manuscript; and Barry Shapiro of the Audio-Visual Unit of the Albert Einstein College of Medicine for preparing several of the figures. While any merits this report may have are in large measure attributable to those who have helped us, any errors of fact or interpretation are the sole responsibility of the authors.

† Dr. Lamm is a resident in pediatrics at the Bronx Municipal Hospital Center, and a member of the Department of Pediatrics at the Albert Einstein College of Medicine.

skepticism about the accomplishments of China's health care system among those in the West who are used to measuring accomplishments in statistical rather than in descriptive terms.

In the wake of the Cultural Revolution, fragmentary statistical data are again beginning to become available. In October 1972 Sidel met at length with representatives of the Shanghai Bureau of Public Health and was provided with the data presented in this paper.* The data must be viewed with caution for several reasons:

1. Definitions used in Shanghai, such as "live births" and "neonatal deaths," and classifications such as causes of death, may not be directly comparable to those used in the United States.

2. Some of the data are based on a three-month collection period—in general too short a time frame to permit adjustment for seasonal or cyclical variations.

3. There are few, and in most cases no, independent ways currently available of ascertaining the completeness or accuracy of the data. This is a problem in interpreting vital statistics collected almost anywhere in the world, but it may be a special handicap in a country where the people needed to gather the information (in contrast to public health leaders) have had little training or experience in assembling statistical data, and may not have a clear perception of the value of reliable data.

4. The statistics for Shanghai are almost certainly not representative of the rest of the country, or even of other large Chinese cities.

One potential criticism we are convinced is *not* justified, however, is that of falsification or manipulation of the data simply to impress a foreign visitor. We were assured, and are convinced, that these are the same figures Shanghai public health officials are using in their own planning and evaluation of programs. As such, the statistics may provide some initial impressions of the state of health of the people of Shanghai and, at the very least, a pre-

* The officials who provided the data were: Dr. Hong Ming-gui, head of the revolutionary committee of the Shanghai Bureau of Public Health, and head of the Shanghai branch of the Chinese Medical Association; Dr. Wang Shi-mong, chief, Department of Curative Medicine, Pharmacy, Hygiene, and Public Health, Shanghai Bureau of Public Health; and Dr. Chiang Lian-yi, member of the department.

liminary baseline with which later data from Shanghai and the rest of China can be compared.

DEMOGRAPHIC STRUCTURE

The Municipality of Shanghai

Shanghai is an independent municipality consisting of ten counties and the city proper, covering 2,250 square miles. The municipality, with a 1972 population estimated at 10.5 million, is located just south of the mouth of the Yangtse River, and borders on the provinces of Kiangsu, of which it was once a part, and Chekiang (Figure 15).

Shanghai City Proper, consisting of ten urban districts covering 54 square miles and encompassing 5.8 million people, is situated on the Whangpoo River, a tributary of the Yangtse (Figure 16). The border between the city proper and the rural counties within the municipality is extremely sharp; one moves from densely settled urban neighborhoods to land used predominantly for agriculture, with no hint of the suburban sprawl that usually separates urban from rural in the United States.

The main commercial area of the city is located on the left bank of the Whangpoo River at the mouth of the Soochow Creek, in what is now the Whangpoo district. Here lie the broad boulevards known in the "bitter past" as the Bund, along the waterfront, now called Chungshan (Dr. Sun Yat-sen) Road, and Nanking Road, with its imposing buildings that used to house foreign banks, shipping houses, and hotels. The major industrial sections include the Hungkow district, north of Soochow Creek, and an area known as Pootung on the right bank of the Whangpoo. The Luwan district, whose recent census is described in the following pages, is an old, mixed, commercial, industrial, and residential district. The Yangpu district, in which we studied a residents' committee, described in detail in Chapter II, is part of the area where there was a spread of urbanization during the 1950s and 1960s along both sides of the Whangpoo toward its mouth at Paoshan on the Yangtse.

In addition to being a large and thriving commercial center,

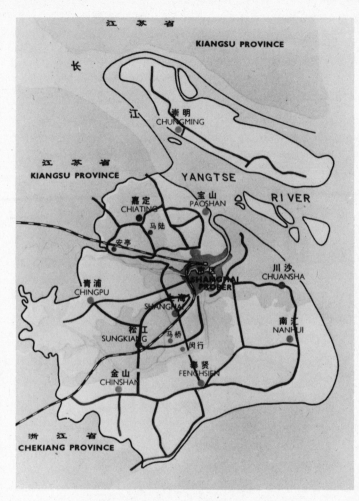

FIGURE 15. Map of Shanghai municipality.

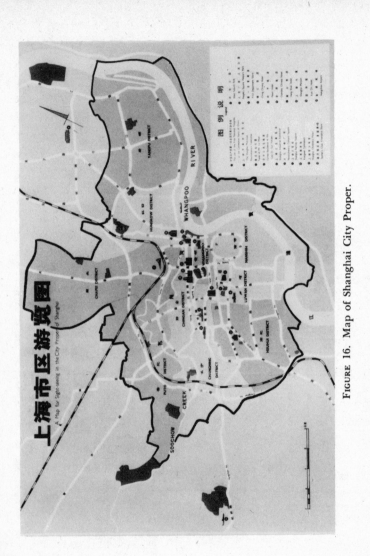

FIGURE 16. Map of Shanghai City Proper.

Shanghai is probably the most flourishing industrial center in China. Over the past two decades the former importance of the city's textile industry declined with the development of heavy industry—iron and steel, chemicals, electrical equipment, heavy machinery, machine tools, and motor vehicles. Nonetheless Shanghai is still the largest textile producer, using not only cotton, wool, and natural silk, but synthetic fiber produced by the city's chemical industry.[3]

Outside the city proper but within the Shanghai municipality there are about 200 communes with a cultivated land area of approximately 1,400 square miles, over half the land area of the ten rural counties. These communes grow mainly rice, wheat, and vegetables to feed the city, and cotton for its mills.

Population Density

The population density of the Shanghai municipality—4,500 people per square mile—is calculated in Table 10. The table also shows the population density of what the United States Bureau of the Census defines as the New York-Northeastern New Jersey

TABLE 10. POPULATION DENSITY: SHANGHAI MUNICIPALITY AND NEW YORK CITY

	Population	Area (Sq. Mi.)	Population Density (Sq. Mi.)
Shanghai			
Entire Municipality	10,500,000	2,350	4,500
City Proper	5,800,000	54	110,000
Outside City Proper	4,700,000	2,296	2,000
New York City			
"Standard Consolidated Area"	16,200,000	3,938	4,100
City Proper	7,900,000	320	25,000
Bronx	1,500,000	41	36,000
Brooklyn	2,600,000	81	32,000
Manhattan	1,500,000	22	69,000
Queens	2,000,000	119	17,000
Richmond	300,000	57	5,200
Outside City Proper	8,300,000	3,618	2,300

"Standard Consolidated Area." This mass of contiguous communities covers a land area about 60 per cent larger than that of the Shanghai municipality; its population is also about 60 per cent larger, leading to a population density—4,100 people per square mile—very similar to that of Shanghai. The areas outside Shanghai City Proper and outside New York City also have remarkably similar population densities. The two great differences of course are that much of the land surrounding New York is "suburban" and used very little for agricultural purposes, and that New York is surrounded by "satellite" cities such as Jersey City, Newark, White Plains, and Yonkers, while only small towns are scattered through Shanghai's surrounding agricultural areas. The relative sizes of the two metropolitan areas may be seen in Figure 17, in which a map of the Shanghai municipality is superimposed on a map of the New York City area drawn to the same scale.

Despite the remarkable similarities of the overall densities of the outer areas, the population density of Shanghai City Proper—110,000 per square mile—is four times that of New York City. The magnitude of this difference can be seen graphically in Figure 18, where a map of Shanghai City Proper has been superimposed on a map of one of New York's five boroughs, the Bronx, drawn to the same scale. Whereas the land area of Shanghai City Proper is about 30 per cent larger than that of the Bronx, its population is about 300 per cent larger. The population density of Shanghai City Proper is therefore about three times that of the Bronx, and about double that of our most tightly packed, major geographic unit, Manhattan Island.

Furthermore the people of Shanghai, with very rare exceptions, live in buildings no higher than five stories, which means that the density is produced by people living in a very small amount of space. Although some investigators have found a correlation between overcrowding and "pathological behavior" in animal populations,* the high population density of Shanghai is said not to be detrimental to the quality of life. While is is possible that with natural increase and immigration the population density may be greater in some areas of the city now than before, the

* The literature on this topic has been reviewed by Galle and his colleagues, who also find evidence for a similar correlation in the city of Chicago.⁴

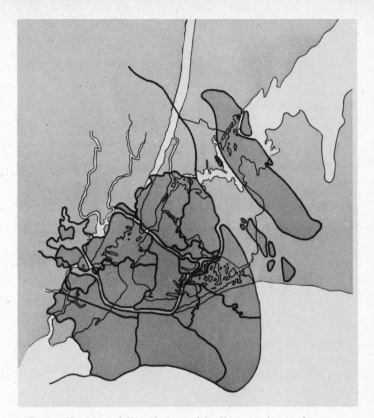

FIGURE 17. Map of Shanghai municipality superimposed on a map of New York City.

residents describe their living conditions as considerably better than before 1949.

Age Distribution

While no recent census has been taken of Shanghai as a whole, one of its ten districts, Luwan, was canvassed in 1971. The Shanghai public health officials say they have no reason to believe that the age distribution of Luwan differs significantly from that of the other urban districts. The age distribution of Luwan's

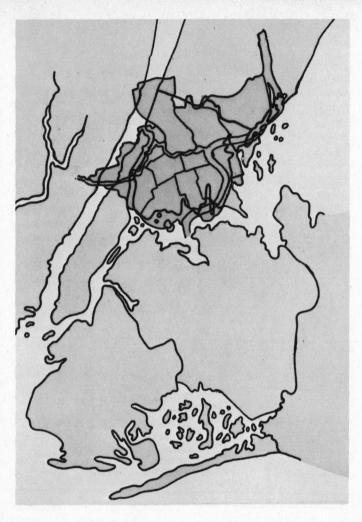

FIGURE 18. Map of Shanghai City Proper superimposed on a map of the Bronx, New York.

population compared to that of the white and nonwhite population of New York City is shown in Table 11. Luwan's population profile, compared with that of the United States, is shown in Figure 19.

A population profile shows the age distribution by a lateral bar representing the percent of the population at each single year of age. Profiles for economically poorly developed societies are generally triangular, with a sharply decreasing percentage at each succeeding year of age. There is a broad base, narrowing, usually rapidly, to a sharp peak due to high birth and mortality rates. The profile for economically developed countries with lower birth and mortality rates, particularly in the younger age groups,

TABLE 11. AGE DISTRIBUTION: LUWAN DISTRICT, SHANGHAI, AND NEW YORK CITY

Age	Approxi-mate Birth-date	Luwan District (1971 Census) Number	%	New York City (1970 Census) White %	Non-white %	Total %
0-4	1966-70	21,762	4.6	7.0	10.5	7.8
5-9	1961-65	36,177	7.6	7.0	11.3	8.0
10-14	1956-60	69,971	14.6	7.1	10.4	7.9
15-19	1951-55	55,382	11.6	7.2	9.0	7.6
20-24	1946-50	32,276	6.7	8.2	8.2	8.2
25-29	1941-45	26,733	5.6	7.3	8.3	7.6
30-34	1936-40	22,900	4.8	5.6	7.5	6.1
35-39	1931-35	35,295	7.4	5.3	6.7	5.6
40-44	1926-30	38,179	8.0	5.9	6.2	6.0
45-49	1921-25	35,155	7.3	6.2	5.6	6.1
50-54	1916-20	28,239	5.9	6.3	4.5	5.8
55-59	1911-15	23,671	5.0	6.6	3.6	5.9
60-64	1906-10	18,879	4.0	6.2	2.9	5.4
65-69	1901-05	15,792	3.3	5.2	2.3	4.5
70-74	1896-1900	9,554	2.0	4.1	1.5	3.4
75-79	1891-95	5,109	1.1	2.6	0.8	2.2
80-84	1886-90	2,113	0.4	1.4	0.4	1.2
85 or over	1885 or earlier	731	0.1	0.8	0.3	0.7
TOTAL		477,918	100.0	100.0	100.0	100.0

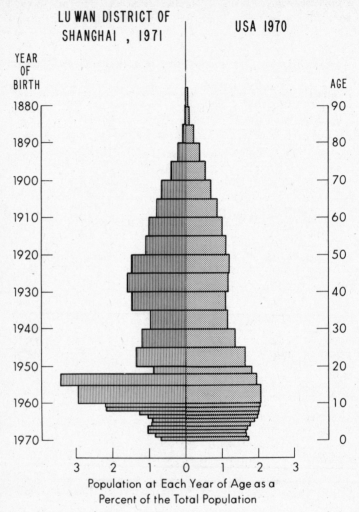

FIGURE 19. Population profiles: Luwan district, Shanghai, and the United States.

is more "rectangular" than "triangular." A typical "traditional" profile (Costa Rica, 1955) and a typical profile for an economically developed country (Sweden, 1956) are shown in Figure 20.[5]

The Luwan profile differs from the "traditional" profile and from the United States and New York City age distribution in a number of aspects, particularly for people under age thirty-five. Indentations in the profile can be explained on the basis of decreased fertility during the years of birth corresponding to a given age group, by selective increased mortality in later years, and by outmigration. Famine, war, and deprivation frequently result in decreased fertility, usually accompanied by an increased infant mortality rate. Other factors causing indentations or bulges

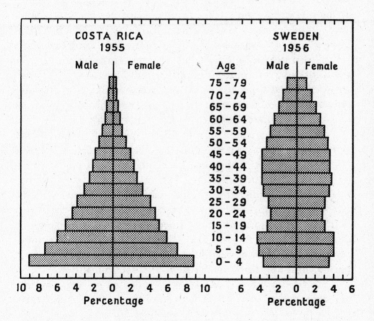

FIGURE 20. Typical population profiles: Costa Rica and Sweden. (Reproduced from Harold F. Dorn, "World Population Growth," in *The Population Dilemma*, ed. P. M. Hauser, © 1963 by the American Assembly, Columbia University. By permission of Prentice-Hall, Inc., Englewood Cliffs, New Jersey.)

include governmental policies on birth control and changes in the availability of certain health care resources such as abortions and contraceptives.

In the Luwan district the eighteen to thirty-five-year age group appears to be under-represented, which may be due to a decreased number of births between 1935 and 1952, to a selective increased mortality in later years, or to selective outmigration. Since the thirty-five- to fifty-year age group does not appear to be under-represented, the relatively low number of those in the eighteen to thirty-five group cannot be explained on the basis of fewer available parents. An explanation of the decrease in fertility in 1935–52 would require evidence that conditions of famine and war were markedly greater in those years than in 1920–35. Reports of the dislocation and social turbulence during the Sino-Japanese and Second World Wars, and the subsequent revolution, support this explanation. Increased childhood mortality during that period would also not be surprising. It is interesting that there is no apparent deficiency in the group that would have been of military age during that time. It should be noted, however, that Luwan is only one district of one city, and that there may have been a selective outmigration of people of working age from that district.*

A great bulge appears in the Luwan profile for children aged eight to eighteen, that is, those born from 1952 to 1962, suggesting a large number of births during this period. This may have had several causes. First, an increase in births is often seen following a severe war, as soldiers return and stability is restored. A second factor in the apparent rise in the birth rate during those years is the increase in the number of people in the fertile age group, those born in the 1920–35 bulge. Third, government policy toward birth control in China vacillated between pro and con during this period, thus appearing inconsistent and ineffective.

In 1950 a new marriage law, intended to end arranged marriages and to give free choice to both men and women, raised

---

* Selective inmigration and outmigration are probably important factors in the current demographic structure of Shanghai. For example, Orleans reports that "during some six months of 1955 that city 'mobilized a total of 555,000 persons for return to the rural areas.' Nevertheless, as people were being moved out, others apparently managed to enter, so that by the middle of 1956 the population of the city reportedly had increased by yet another half million." [6]

the marriage age to eighteen for women and to twenty for men. In April 1952 Peking's *Jenmin Ribao* (*People's Daily*), calling birth control "a means of killing off the Chinese people without shedding blood," denounced it on the grounds that people are "the most precious of all categories of capital." [7] From 1954 to 1957 public policy encouraged birth control in order to make more women available for productive work and child health care. In 1958, the year of the Great Leap Forward, an anti-birth-control policy was frequently enunciated. This was succeeded by three years of economic crisis during which there was little mention of birth control, either pro or con. These fluctuations in public policy are not specifically mirrored in the population profile for Luwan, which suggests a high birth rate throughout the period 1952–62.

By 1962 public policy was once more encouraging limitation of family size. Except for a short time during the Cultural Revolution when birth control programs were ignored, public policy included the intensive propagation of "planned birth." This effort, which also urged late marriages and small families, was intensified in the past few years, particularly in the cities. The median age at first parity is as yet unknown, but it is almost certainly growing later, with women being urged to delay marriage until age twenty-four to twenty-six, and men until twenty-six to twenty-nine. This delay in the age of first parity, if it results in a greater median age of parity, will increase the generation interval; it may also lead to smaller family size. The Luwan profile appears to reflect the fall in urban birth rates— less than 5 per cent of the population is under the age of four, compared to 7 per cent of the white and almost 11 per cent of the nonwhite populations in that age group in New York City.

One additional facet of the age profile is the relative dearth of elderly people in Luwan compared to the white population of New York City and to the entire population of the United States, but not in comparison to the nonwhite New York City population. This may reflect famine and pestilence in earlier periods. Another hypothesis explaining this difference would be the poor medical care available early in the lives of Luwan's older people, resulting in the deaths of a number of them, and possibly relatively poor care for the older population compared to that for the younger after 1950. This latter aspect may be supported by the age-specific death rates. In the older age group the age-specific death rates for Shanghai exceed those of both Sweden and the New York City white population. A much more likely explanation, however, is selective inmigration and outmigration. For example, young white people often leave their parents behind when they move from New York City to the suburbs; those moving into the city, on the other hand, mainly blacks and Puerto Ricans, are for the most part quite young. Thus one need not invoke differential health or health care patterns—although they surely exist—to explain the difference.

BIRTH RATES

Crude Birth Rate

The crude birth rate in Shanghai City Proper may be calculated from the data provided by the Bureau of Public Health for January through March 1972, when there were 8,662 live births in Shanghai's ten urban districts. Assuming that January to March are typical birth months—an assumption unlikely to be fully correct—total annual births in Shanghai City Proper would be about 35,000. The 1971 estimates of the population of Shanghai City Proper given us by the bureau was 5,697,800, leading to an annual crude birth rate of 6.1 per 1,000 population, which is almost unbelievably low, compared to a New York City 1970 rate of 17.1 per 1,000 for whites and 24.7 for nonwhites (Table 12). The rate for the United States as a whole in 1970 was 18.2 per 1,000, the lowest, 15.5 per 1,000, being in the state of Maryland. West Berlin has a reported rate of 9.5 per 1,000, in comparison with 13.3 in the Federal Republic of Germany; Sweden and Finland both have rates of 13.7; the rates for Stockholm and Helsinki can reasonably be assumed to be on the order of 10.

What is most astonishing is not the comparison of the Shanghai City Proper birth rate with those of cities in relatively richer countries, but with those in other poorer countries of

TABLE 12. CRUDE BIRTH AND DEATH RATES: SHANGHAI CITY PROPER
AND NEW YORK CITY

	Shanghai [a]	New York City [b]	
		White	Nonwhite
Crude birth rate [c]	6.1	17.1	24.7
Crude death rate [d]	6.4	12.1	8.1
Natural growth rate [e]	−0.3	5.0	16.6

Notes: (a) Extrapolated from data for January through March 1972; (b) data
for 1970; (c) births per 1,000 population per year; (d) deaths per 1,000 population
per year; (e) change in population per 1,000 population per year. Extrapolation to
an entire year on the basis of three-month data is risky; visitors in 1973 have been
given the figure of about 0.8 per 1,000 for the natural population increase for
Shanghai City Proper for all of 1972.

Asia * as well as with other areas of China. While Southeast Asia
as a whole is reported by the United Nations to have a crude
birth rate of 43 per 1,000, China's estimated rate is approximately
30 per 1,000. Even the Shanghai counties have a considerably
higher rate—approximately 18 births per 1,000—than does the
city proper.

If the age distribution for Luwan is indeed typical of the
city as a whole, one factor that helps Shanghai to maintain its
low rate is the relatively small percentage of its population in
the fertile age group.† Women born during the huge birth spurt
from 1952 to 1960 are just now entering their childbearing
years, so Shanghai's crude birth rate is almost certain to rise
over the next few years. Predictions of the magnitude of the
increase would require knowledge of current fertility rates, of
projected changes in them, and of other factors not yet avail-

* Such comparisons must be viewed with suspicion since the number of births
in developing countries is usually under-reported and then corrected for estimated
error.

† It is impossible to calculate a fertility rate for Shanghai since specific data
on the number of women in the childbearing years are not yet available. The best
estimate that can be made from the data provided requires the assumption that
the percent of the population aged fifteen to forty-four in Shanghai City Proper
is the same as in Luwan district (44.1 percent), and, furthermore, that half of this
group is female. These assumptions lead to an estimate of 1,256,000 women aged
fifteen to forty-four in Shanghai City Proper. The calculated general fertility rate
is therefore 35,000:1,256,000, or 28 births per 1,000; the comparable United States
rate for 1970 is 88.

able. Whether Shanghai's birth control efforts can prevent a
sharp rise in the birth rate will provide an important test of
the efficiency of the program.

Plural Births

The 8,662 babies born alive in Shanghai City Proper in the
first three months of 1972 were born to 8,622 women. We have
no data on how many of these birth events were twins, triplets,
or other multiples, but for the purpose of initial calculations
we will assume that all the multiple births were twins, and
that there were not a significant number of multiple births in
which one baby was born alive and one dead. Based on these
assumptions, there were forty pairs of twins born during this
period, or eighty "plural births." Thus the plural birth ratio
(plural live births: total live births) was 9.0 per 1,000 live births
(80:8,662).

This is considerably less than United States ratios of 19.4
for white babies and 23.8 for nonwhite babies. A recent study in
Taiwan showed a plural birth ratio of 20.9.* This would suggest
that the apparently low ratio for Shanghai City Proper is not
due to genetic differences in twinning frequencies between
Chinese and Americans. Furthermore, since in the United States
the frequency of twinning rises with maternal age, and since the
median age at parity in Shanghai is almost certainly higher than
that in the United States, one would have predicted the frequency of twinning to be higher in Shanghai than in the United
States.

The profound difference in plural birth ratio may be due to
differences in classification (for example, women delivering stillborns may have been included in the total of women delivering
during the period) † or due to incomplete reporting of live borns

* In this study, performed in six hospitals over a three-year period, there were
25,090 live-born single births, 258 twin sets, and seven sets of triplets, for a total of
25,627 live borns, of which 537 were plural births.[8] The calculation 537:25,627 leads
to a plural birth ratio of 20.9:1,000, very similar to the ratio in the United States.
Furthermore if one takes the total live borns (25,627) and the total women delivered
of live babies (25.355) in this study, and performs a calculation using the same
assumptions we used in dealing with Shanghai data, the plural birth ratio is 544:
25,627 or 21.2:1,000, almost indistinguishable from the true ratio.
† This error of inclusion of all mothers of stillborns in the total of women

at the time the data were given to us. Since studies of twinning
in many countries have shown a rather consistent monozygotic
twinning rate of 7–9 (3.5–4.5) per 1,000 live births,[10] the data
implies an almost complete elimination of dizygotic twins, which
is improbable. It is more likely that the data, or our intrepreta-
tion of them, are in some way in error. But if the difference
in plural birth ratios between Shanghai and elsewhere is real and
sustained, its explanation will be intriguing and important.

MORTALITY

Crude Death Rate

For the three months, January through March 1972, the
total number of deaths in Shanghai City Proper was reported as
9,142. Again making the assumption that deaths are evenly distributed over the calendar year, which is even more suspect than
the comparable assumption for births, (in the United States,
deaths are more common in the winter),* there would have been
36,568 deaths among the 5,697,800 inhabitants. Thus the calculated crude death rate is 6.4 per 1,000 people annually.

The fact that the crude death rate in Shanghai City Proper
is considerably lower than the New York City rate (Table 3),
is as much or more due to the different age structure of the
Shanghai population as it is to the age-specific death rates to be
discussed later. This is illustrated by the New York City nonwhite crude death rate (8.1) being lower than the white rate

---

delivering is not likely. For example, data published by the National Center for
Health Statistics for 1964 permit the calculation for the United States of the
3,987,000 women delivering the 4,027,500 live born infants in that year.[9] Thus use
of these two numbers, and the assumptions used for Shanghai, lead to the calculation of a plural birth ratio of 20.1 per 1,000, very close to the "true" ratio. If the
number of reported stillbirths at twenty-eight weeks and over in 1964 (43,400) is
added to the number of women delivering live borns, the total number of women
delivering (4,030,400) *exceeds* the number of live born babies. If the ratio of reported
stillbirths to live births in Shanghai is similar to the United States ratio, this would
rule out the inclusion of *all* women delivering stillborns in the total of women
delivering. On the other hand, an error may lie in the inclusion in the Shanghai
total of *some* women delivering stillborns.

* There is some evidence that this is also true in Shanghai; in another context
we were given the deaths for Shanghai City Proper from January to June 1972 as
15,717 (Table 14). Thus there appear to have been only 6,575 deaths reported from
April through June 1972. The six-month total doubled leads to an estimated crude
death rate of 5.5 per 1,000 people.

(12.1), despite the fact that the nonwhite age-specific rate is higher at almost every age than the white rate; this statistical anomaly is due to a greater percentage of nonwhites in the lower age groups, where death rates are lower. The crude death rate for the entire Shanghai municipality is even lower, 5.9 per 1,000, probably reflecting a higher percentage of younger people in the Shanghai counties than in its urban districts.

The importance of the crude death rate lies in comparing it with the crude birth rate. Based on these data (Table 12), Shanghai may have transiently achieved negative natural population increase, a stage the United States is not likely to reach for several decades, despite the rapid fall in its fertility rate. Again, however, the point must be made that the growth rate in Shanghai City Proper, measured over a full year, is positive— approximately 0.8 per 1,000—and will probably increase when the large group of people born between 1952 and 1962 reach the age of parenthood.

Infant Mortality Rates

The data provided by the Bureau of Public Health shows 109 deaths under one year of age in Shanghai City Proper during the first three months of 1972. From this may be calculated an infant death rate of 12.6 per 1,000 live births. The number of deaths within thirty days of birth was reported as twenty-eight, leading to a calculated neonatal death rate of 3.2 per 1,000 live births.* These rates are compared with New York City rates in Table 13.

The difference in the neonatal death rates is extraordinary. Shanghai's rate might be explained on the basis of the prevention of birth of high-risk infants and improved prenatal or neonatal death, or by erroneous data collection or reporting. It may be, for example, that differences in contraceptive patterns and in prenatal and obstetrical care in China and the United States have led to differences in the incidence of such risk factors as prematurity, "small-for-dates" babies, and/or respiratory disease syndromes, but such data are not yet available.

---

* In the United States, as in most other countries, the standard definition used for the "neonatal" period is twenty-eight rather than thirty days.

TABLE 13. INFANT DEATH RATES: SHANGHAI CITY PROPER
AND NEW YORK CITY

(Per 1,000 Live Births)

	Shanghai [a]	New York City [b] White	Nonwhite
Infant death rates (Under one year of age)	12.6	18.1	27.1
Neonatal death rates (Within 28 days [U.S.] or 30 days [Shanghai])	3.2	13.4	18.6
Postneonatal death rates (Deaths in remainder of first year of life)	9.4	4.7	8.5
Neonatal deaths as a percentage of total infant deaths	25.7	74.0	68.6

Notes: (a) Data for January through March 1972; (b) data for 1971.

Even if all these factors are taken into consideration, however, the low neonatal death rate is most remarkable, particularly
since the postneonatal death rate in Shanghai appears to considerably exceed that of New York City. Neonatal deaths usually
account for most infant deaths—in New York City they now
account for 74 per cent of white infant deaths; the Shanghai data
indicate they account for only 24 per cent of infant deaths. It is
possible that through a misunderstanding the figures for neonatal deaths and postneonatal deaths were reversed.* If this

* Another possible explanation is that "live birth" is not defined, or the definition is not applied in the same way, in Shanghai as in the United States or in
other countries, and that some babies who die shortly after birth are counted neither
as live births nor infant deaths, but as stillbirths; this would lead to an under-
statement of both the neonatal and total infant mortality rates, and to a very
slight overestimate of the postneonatal rates. Further exploration of this possibility
will have to await the opportunity to examine the definition and its application
in Shanghai in detail. For comparability with other nations it is to be hoped that
China has adopted, or will adopt, the definition of live birth adopted by the Third
World Health Assembly in 1950: "Live birth is the complete expulsion or extraction
from its mother of a product of conception, irrespective of the duration of pregnancy,

were so, the data would be more consistent, in that both the neonatal and the postneonatal death rates in Shanghai would be about 70 per cent that of white babies in New York City. Such a reversal of the data would also make the percent of neonatal deaths in Shanghai (74.3) almost precisely the same as that among whites in New York City (74.0).

Assuming that the total infant mortality rate of 12.6 per 1,000 for Shanghai City Proper is indeed correct, or correct to within 10 to 20 per cent, it is remarkably low. This is true not only in comparison with New York City or the United States as a whole,* but even more so in comparison with infant mortality rates of countries at a stage of technological development comparable to that of China. Among the countries of Southeast Asia, for example, Indonesia and Cambodia have rates of 125 per 1,000 live births—ten times the reported rate for Shanghai; India's rate is 139. It should be noted, however, that the same limitations on the data discussed for birth rates apply to infant mortality rates, and that it is of course improper for most purposes to compare rates for a city with those for an entire country.

Age-Specific Death Rates

The infant mortality rate is a special example of an age-specific death rate—a much more useful tool for determining the health of a population than the crude death rate. The Bureau of Public Health was able to provide the numerators for the calculation of age-specific rates, that is, the number of deaths in Shanghai City Proper in each age group over the six-month period, January through June 1972; it could not, however, pro-

---

which, after such separation breathes or shows any other evidence of life, such as beating of the heart, pulsation of the umbilical cord, or definite movement of voluntary muscles, whether or not the umbilical cord has been cut or the placenta is attached; each product of such a birth is considered live born." [11]

* It is of interest that in 1968 the "white" infant death rate in the United States was 19.2 per 1,000, and that for "other races" 34.5, while in the state of Hawaii, which has the lowest rates, it was 15.6 per 1,000 for white babies and 19.2 for those of other races. Rates as low as those for Shanghai have been reported for selected low-risk groups; for example, a recent study of births in New York City in 1968 shows an infant death rate of 9.4 for "foreign-born white women with no extra medical or social risks." [12]

vide the denominator, the population in the city proper for each age group. We have therefore projected the population in each age group in the city proper from the age distribution of the Luwan district and the total population of the city; this procedure assumes of course that the age distribution of Luwan is similar to that of the whole city, an assumption the bureau thought reasonable. A further assumption is that a doubling of deaths in that six-month period is a good approximation of the annual death rate. The data for the calculation of age-specific death rates and the rates themselves are shown in Table 14.

These rates are compared with those of the New York City

TABLE 14. CALCULATION OF AGE-SPECIFIC DEATH RATES:
SHANGHAI CITY PROPER

Age	Number of Deaths [a]	Estimated Population in Each Age Group [b]	Age-Specific Death Rates [c]
Less than 1	183	39,544	.009255
1	31	48,319	.001283
2	25	59,487	.000840
3	17	59,202	.000574
4	10	52,877	.000378
5-9	63	431,279	.000292
10-14	106	834,244	.000254
15-19	180	660,284	.000545
20-29	295	703,531	.000838
30-39	499	693,845	.001438
40-49	1,247	874,357	.002852
50-59	2,372	618,915	.007665
60-69	4,159	413,332	.020124
70-79	4,396	174,814	.050293
80 and over	2,134	33,901	.125895
Total	15,717	5,697,931	.005517

Notes: (a) Data for January through June 1972; (b) age distribution for Shanghai City Proper projected from census of Luwan district, 1971; (c) deaths in 6 months in age group X2
Population in age group .

white and nonwhite populations and the population of Sweden *
(Figure 21). It may be seen that, with few exceptions, at any
specific age the risk of dying is greater for a nonwhite than a
white New Yorker, greater for a white New Yorker than a resident of Shanghai, and greater for a Shanghai resident than a
Swedish citizen. The graph of the age-specific death rates for
Shanghai indicates that at all ages the city's health indices are
similar to those of the highly technologically developed areas
of the world.

The low rate in children aged two to fifteen is indicative
of the control of malnutrition and of the usual childhood
diseases, including gastroenteritis, which in the past were said to
have caused a large proportion of childhood deaths in Shanghai.
Other childhood deaths are due to accidents; in the United
States accidents are responsible for more deaths than any other
cause in the age group between one and twenty years.

In later years the differences in age-specific death rates are
largely due to preventable causes—accidents, homicides, suicides,
and premature deaths from degenerative diseases such as hypertension, diabetes, and heart disease. In the age group twenty to
fifty, the age-specific death rates for white and nonwhite New
Yorkers are greater than for both Shanghai and Sweden, with
New York nonwhite rates very much higher. Although some
deaths in this age group are as yet "unpreventable"—deaths from
malignancy or hereditary disease for example—differences in
mortality rates in this group are thought to reflect the general
environmental and social health of the population.[13]

In the groups over age fifty the major causes of death are
heart disease, cancer, and stroke. Nonetheless, differences in age-
specific death rates among the elderly may reflect the attention
paid to care for the aged, as well as disease incidence and genetic
propensities.

---

* While it is, as we have stated, quite improper for most purposes to compare
death rates for a country with those for a city, Sweden's data are used simply as an
example of extremely low death rates.

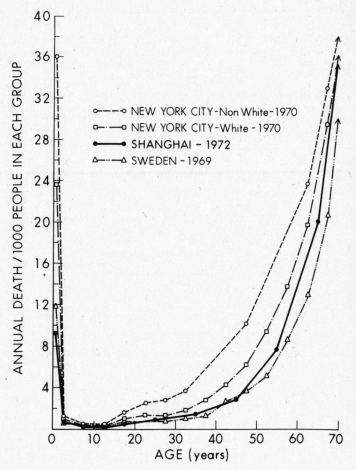

FIGURE 21. Age-specific death rates: Shanghai, New York City, and Sweden.

Leading Causes of Death

The leading causes of death in Shanghai City Proper for January–June 1972 are shown in Tables 15 and 16, where they are compared with the leading causes of death in the United States and New York City, respectively. Since it is very likely that causes of death are ascribed quite differently in Shanghai than in the United States (for example, "old age" is used as a category in Shanghai), the percentage figures must be approached with great caution. Nonetheless, two points are striking:

1. As in the technologically highly developed countries, the degenerative diseases of older people predominate as the causes of death. This is reported to be a marked change for Shanghai, where only two decades ago the leading causes of death were said to be the sequellae of malnutrition and infectious disease.

TABLE 15. CAUSES OF DEATH: SHANGHAI CITY PROPER
AND THE UNITED STATES

Shanghai (January–June 1972)	%	United States (1968)	%
1. Cancer	25.3	Cardiovascular disease	38.7
2. Cerebrovascular disease	19.3	Cancer	16.5
3. Cardiovascular disease	12.1	Cerebrovascular disease	11.0
4. Respiratory disease	8.4	Accidents	6.0
5. Old age *	8.3	Influenza and pneumonia	3.8
6. Digestive disease	6.1	Certain diseases of early infancy	2.3
7. Accidents	4.9	Diabetes mellitus	2.0
8. Lung disease	4.1	Arteriosclerosis	1.7
9. Pneumonia	2.2	Lung: emphysema, bronchitis, asthma	1.7
10. Kidney disease	1.7	Cirrhosis of liver	1.5
All others	7.6	All others	14.8
TOTAL	100.0		100.0

* This category is not used in the United States. Causes 1, 2, 3, and 5 together account for 65 per cent of the deaths in Shanghai; causes 1, 2, and 3 account for 66.2 per cent of the deaths in the United States.

TABLE 16. CAUSES OF DEATH: SHANGHAI CITY PROPER
AND NEW YORK CITY

| | Shanghai [a] | New York City [b] | |
| | | White | Nonwhite |
	%	%	%
Cancer	25	23	18
Stroke	19	7	· 8
Heart disease	12	45	28
All others	44	25	46
Total	100	100	100

Notes: (a) Data for January through June 1972; (b) data for 1970.

2. Although heart disease, cancer, and stroke appear to be the three leading causes of death in both Shanghai and the United States, their rank order differs. In the United States, and among New York City whites and nonwhites, heart disease is followed by cancer and stroke; in Shanghai heart disease is only the third leading cause, preceded by cancer and stroke.

Both of these points deserve detailed further exploration as they are of great significance in the provision of preventive and therapeutic medical care in both China and the United States.

LIFE TABLE AND LIFE EXPECTANCY

Life tables, and the "life expectancies" derived from them, artificial devices used to compare death rates among different populations, are calculated from age-specific death rates. An estimated abridged life table, constructed from the Shanghai data with the assistance of Robert J. Armstrong of the National Center for Health Statistics, is given in Table 17. An explanation of the derivation of each column may be found, for example, in Barclay's *Techniques of Population Analysis*.[14]

Finally, Table 18 compares the life expectancies at each age for Shanghai with those for the United States. For each age until the seventh decade, the life expectancy is greater in Shanghai than in the United States. Based on the still limited data, the

TABLE 17. ESTIMATED ABRIDGED LIFE TABLE FOR SHANGHAI CITY PROPER

Age in Years	Age Specific Death Rate $_nm_x$	Probability of Dying during Age Interval $_nq_x$	Survivors Entering Interval l_x	Number of Deaths during Interval $_nd_x$	Years Lived during Interval $_nL_x$	Total Years Lived after Entering Interval T_x	Life Expectancy (Average Number of Years Lived by Persons after Entering Age Interval) e_x
Less than 1	.009255	.008454	100,000	845	99,282	7,331,142	73.3
1-4	.000755	.003014	99,155	299	395,872	7,231,860	72.9
5-9	.000292	.001459	98,856	144	493,920	6,835,988	69.2
10-14	.000254	.001269	98,712	125	493,248	6,342,068	64.2
15-19	.000545	.002721	98,587	268	492,265	5,848,820	59.3
20-29	.000838	.008345	98,319	820	979,090	5,356,555	54.5
30-39	.001438	.014277	97,499	1,392	968,030	4,377,465	44.9
40-49	.002852	.028119	96,107	2,702	947,560	3,409,435	35.5
50-59	.007665	.073821	93,405	6,895	899,575	2,461,875	26.4
60-69	.020124	.182842	86,510	15,818	786,010	1,562,300	18.1
70-79	.050293	.401873	70,692	28,409	564,875	776,290	11.0
80 and over	.125895	1.000000	42,283	42,283	211,415	211,415	5.0

TABLE 18. LIFE EXPECTANCY: SHANGHAI CITY PROPER
AND THE UNITED STATES

Age in Years	Shanghai (1972)	United States (1969)
	e_x	e_x
Less than 1	73.3	70.4
1-4	72.9	71.0
5-9	69.2	67.2
10-14	64.2	62.3
15-19	59.3	57.5
20-29	54.5	52.8
30-39	44.9	43.5
40-49	35.5	34.3
50-59	26.4	25.7
60-69	18.1	18.1
70-79	11.0	11.8
80 and over	5.0	7.0

life expectancy at birth in Shanghai now appears to be 73.3 years compared with 70.4 years in the United States. Only from age 70 on is life expectancy greater in the United States.

SUMMARY

Data provided by the Shanghai Bureau of Public Health for early 1972, while fragmentary, yield preliminary health indices similar to those of the technologically highly developed areas of the world. If these data are confirmed by future data, and are found to be based on definitions comparable to those used in other countries, they suggest in statistical terms a highly favorable health profile for the city of Shanghai. They cannot, however, be taken as representative of the country as a whole, or even of other large cities in China.

Many observers have described the visible changes in Shanghai over the past twenty-five years—from the gross evidence of widespread illness and early death from malnutrition and infectious disease in the late 1940s to the picture of vibrant health seen in the 1970s. By separate pathways both the statistician and the observer seem to have arrived at much the same conclusion: Shanghai's residents seem remarkably healthy. This represents a major accomplishment that may well be unprecedented for a country at China's stage of technological development.

NOTES

1. Leo A. Orleans, "China's Statistics: The System and Its Problems," *Public Data Use* 1, no. 2 (April 1973): 17-23.

2. Amaury de Riencourt, *The Soul of China* (New York: Coward McCann, 1958).

3. Theodore Shabad, *China's Changing Map*, rev. ed. (New York: Praeger Publishers, 1972): pp. 136-38.

4. Omer R. Galle, Walter R. Grove, and J. Miller McPherson, "Population Density and Pathology: What Are the Relations for Man?" *Science* 176 (1972): 23-30.

5. Harold F. Dorn, "World Population Growth," in *The Population Dilemma*, ed. P. H. Hauser (Englewood Cliffs, N.J.: Prentice-Hall, 1963).

6. Leo A. Orleans, *Every Fifth Child* (Stanford: Stanford University Press, 1972): p. 64.

7. ———, "China: Population in the People's Republic," *Population Bulletin* 27, no. 6 (1971): 5-37.

8. Irvin Emanuel et al., "The Incidence of Congenital Malformations in a Chinese Population: The Taipei Collaborative Study," *Teratology* 5 (1972): 159-70.

9. *Multiple Births United States—1964, Vital and Health Statistics*, ser. 21, no. 14 (Washington, D.C.: National Center for Health Statistics, 1967).

10. I. H. Porter, *Heredity and Disease* (New York: McGraw-Hill, 1968): p. 293.

11. *International Comparison of Perinatal and Infant Mortality: The United States and Six West European Countries, Vital and Health Statistics*, ser. 3, no. 6 (Washington, D.C.: National Center for Health Statistics, 1967).

12. Harold M. Schmeck, Jr., "Infant Deaths Tied to Poor Health Care," *New York Times* (July 8, 1967).

13. Alex M. Burgess, Jr., Theodore Colton, and Osler L. Peterson, "Categorical Programs for Heart Disease, Cancer and Stroke: Lessons from International Death-Rate Comparisons," *New England Journal of Medicine* 273, no. 10 (September 2, 1965): 533-37.

14. George W. Barclay, *Techniques of Population Analysis* (New York: John Wiley, 1958).

Staff Members of Shoutu (Capital) Hospital,
Peking, September 1972

Revolutionary Committee
Chairman: Pai Hsi-ching, pathologist (on leave because of illness)
Vice-Chairman: Hsieh Hsin-pin, pediatrician
Responsible member, professional group: Yang Sze-pin

Directors of Departments
Dermatology: Li Hung-chua
ENT: Chang Ch'ing-sung
Gynecology and Obstetrics: Lin Ch'iao-chih * (whose name was transliterated in the past as Lim Kha-t'i); deputy director, Ho Tso-hua.
Isotopes: Chou Chien
Laboratory: Li Lin
Medicine: Chang Hsiao-ch'ien * (Cheng Ch'ao-chien)
Neurology: Huang Hui-peng (acting director)
Ophthalmology: Wu Chen
Pediatrics: Chou Hua-kong
Physical Therapy: Yang Sze-pin
Radiology: Hu Mao-hua
Stomatology: Wang Chiao-chang
Surgery: Tseng Hsien-chou; deputy directors, Hsu Lo-tien and Wu Wei-jan; Wu Chieh-ping, deputy director of the Chinese Academy of Medical Science, is on the staff of the urology section.
Traditional Chinese Medicine: Hsih Chi-chiao

* Dr. Lin has been head of the Department of Gynecology and Obstetrics, and Dr. Chang head of the Department of Medicine since the nationalization of PUMC in 1951.

Whereabouts of Former Staff Members *

    Chu Hsien-i (Medicine)—Left to become dean of Tientsin Medical College, and is now an endocrinologist in the Department of Medicine at the college.

    Liu Shih-hao (Medicine)—Still in the Department of Medicine but on sick leave.

    Chu Fu-t'ang (Pediatrics)—Now head of the Peking Children's Hospital.

    Hsieh Chih-kuang (Radiology)—Left to work in Kwangchow, but has since died of cancer.

    Hu Cheng-hsiang (Pathology)—Left to work in the Academy of Medical Sciences, but has since died.

    Samuel H. Zia (Bacteriology)—Now working in the Peking Tumor Hospital of the Academy of Medical Sciences.

    Chang Hsi-chun (Physiology)—Worked in Szechwan for a period but has now returned to Peking, where he is head of physiology in the Academy of Medical Sciences.

    Ch'iu Tsu-yuan (Public Health)—Now at the Peking Tuberculosis Research Institute, located in one of the counties of the Peking municipality.

    Yu Sung-t'ing (Urology)—Now director of surgery, Tientsin Medical College.

    Wu Ying-k'ai (Surgery)—Now head of cardiac surgery at the Fu Wai Hospital of the Academy of Medical Sciences

* Dr. John Z. Bowers of the Macy Foundation gave us the names of these former Peking Union Medical College faculty members, whom he had mentioned in his book, *Western Medicine in a Chinese Palace, Peking Union Medical College, 1917-1951* (New York: Josiah Macy, Jr. Foundation, 1973). Our hosts in China were kind enough to supply the information as to the present whereabouts of these individuals.

"Standard Items" in a Worker Doctor's Medicine
Cabinet and in a Barefoot Doctor's Bag [1]

Medications

Adona ampules (probably an extract of *Adonis versalis,* used as
a cardiac stimulant)

"Adrenalin" (epinephrine) ampules

Aminophyllin tablets and ampules *

Ammonium chloride tablets and solution #

Analgin tablets and ampules (Analgin is the name in the Soviet
Union for the sodium 4-methylaminomethane sulfonate de-
rivative of antipyrine, also known as novalgin; it is an analgesic used for treatment of painful musculoskeletal conditions)

APC (aspirin-phenacetin-caffeine) tablets *#

Atropine tablets

Belladonna extract tablets*#

Berberine tablets * (a traditional Chinese medicine with anti-
biotic properties, probably an alkaloid derived from *Hydrasis
canadensis*)

Brown's mixture tablets and liquid *

"Butazolidin" (phenylbutazone) tablets

Caffeine sodium benzoate ampules

"Chloromycetin" (chloramphenicol) ampules and capsules

Chlorpheniramine maleate tablets #

Chlorpromazine tablets and ampules *# (also known in China
as wintermin and "thorazine")

Chlothamine tablets

"Coramine" (nikethamide) ampules

DCT tablets

"Dolantin" (meperidine) ampules

---

[1] Source: List provided us by Dr. Hsu Chia-yu in October 1971.

* Items found in the bag of a barefoot doctor in a commune outside Peking.

Items found in the cabinet of a worker doctor in a Peking factory.

270

SERVE THE PEOPLE

DPP tablets
Ephedrine sulfate tablets
"Furadantin" (nitrofurantoin) tablets #
Furazolidone tablets *#
Gastropin (8-p-phenylbenzylatropinium bromide) tablets # (a
  ganglionic blocking agent used for the treatment of peptic
  ulcer)
Lobodura tablets
"Luminal" (phenobarbital) tablets *
Paperazine tablets (possibly piperazine citrate, an antihelmin-
  thic)
Penicillin, crystalline
Penicillin, procaine
"Phenergan" (promethazine) tablets
Phenolax tablets *# (a laxative)
"Probanthine" (propantheline bromide) tablets
Reserpine tablets
Sodium bicarbonate tablets
Sulfadiazine tablets and ampules * (also known as SD)
Sulfaguanidine tablets (also known as SG)
Sulfamethazine tablets (also known as SM2)
Sulfamethoxpyridazine tablets *# (also known as SMP)
Sulfathiazole tablets (also known as ST)
Syntomycin capsules (also known as sintomycin)
"Terramycin" (oxtetracycline) tablets
Tetracycline tablets *
"Valium" (diazepam) tablets *
Violactyl (lactobacillus) tablets *
Vitamin B1 tablets *
Vitamin B2 tablets #
Vitamin C tablets #
Vitamin K tablets #
Vitamin U tablets #
Yeast tablets *

Topical Agents
Alcohol *
Boric acid ointment

"Eye drops"
Gentian violet *
Iodine tincture
Mercurochrome *
"Nose drops"
"Sulfa ointment"

Traditional and Herb Medicine
Pills and tablets: type depends on the individual commune or
other unit. Examples include antipyretics *#, antitussives *#,
antispasmodics *#, and medication for dysmenorrhea #.

Equipment
Acupuncture needles *
Adhesive tape
Bandages and gauze
Bowl for changing dressings
Cotton sponges
Cotton swabs *
Drinking cups
Forceps
Fountain pen
Hypodermic needles *
Manometer (sphygmomanometer)
Notebook for records
Paper bag
Rubber tubing
Scissors
Syringes, 2 cc. and 5 cc.*
Thermometers, oral and rectal *

Summary of the Contents of a
Barefoot Doctor's Handbook

Chapter I. Recognition of the Human Body
Section 1—Perceptive Organ System
   Eye; ear; nose; tongue; throat; pharynx
Section 2—Histology of the Skin
Section 3—Nervous System
   Cranial nerves; spinal cord and spinal nerves; autonerves; reflexes
Section 4—Endocrine System
   Thyroid glands; adrenals; insulin; pituitary; gonads
Section 5—Motor System
Section 6—Circulatory System
Section 7—Respiratory System
Section 8—Digestive System
Section 9—Urinary System
Section 10—Reproductive System
Section 11—Characteristics of the Different Systems in Children
Section 12—Perception of the Human Body by Traditional Methods

Chapter II. Common Sense of Hygiene
Section 1—The Patriotic Health Movement
   Water hygiene; management of night soil; food hygiene
Section 2—Hygiene in Agricultural and Industrial Production
Section 3—Wiping Out Pests
   Eradication of flies, mosquitoes, rats, etc.
Section 4—Personal Hygiene
   Oral hygiene; skin and clothing

Medical Colleges in the People's Republic of China

Municipalities	1957 [1]	1964 [2]	1972 [3]
Peking	Peking Medical College	Peking Medical College	Peking Medical College [4]
	Peking College of Chinese Medicine	Peking Chinese Medical College	Peking College of Traditional Chinese Medicine
	—	Peking Military Medical University [5]	No information [5]
	—	China Medical University [6]	No longer functioning as a medical college [6]
	—	—	Peking Second Medical College [7]
Shanghai	Shanghai Medical College No. 1	Shanghai First Medical College	Shanghai First Medical College
	Shanghai Medical College No. 2	Shanghai Second Medical College	Shanghai Second Medical College
	Shanghai College of Chinese Medicine	Shanghai Chinese Medical College	Shanghai College of Traditional Chinese Medicine [8]

Municipalities	*1957*[1]	*1964*[2]	*1972*[3]
	—	Shanghai Railway Medical College	Shanghai Railway Medical College[9]
	—	Shanghai Military Medical University	Shanghai Military Medical University[5]
Tientsin	Tientsin Medical College	Tientsin Medical University	Tientsin Medical College
Provinces[10]	*1957*	*1964*	*1972*
Anhwei	Anhwei Medical College (in Hofei)	Anhwei Medical College	Anhwei Medical College
Chekiang	Chekiang Medical College (in Hangchow)	Chekiang Medical College	Chekiang Medical College
	—	Chekiang Medical University	No information
Fukien	Fukien Medical College (in Foochow)	Fukien Medical College	Fukien Medical University
	—	Fukien Chinese Medical College	(Merged with above in 1969)
Heilungkiang	Harbin Medical College	Harbin Medical University	Harbin Medical University
Honan	Honan Medical College (in Kaifeng)	Honan Medical College (moved to Chengchow)	Honan Medical College
	—	Honan Chinese Medical College	Honan College of Traditional Chinese Medicine

Province			
Hopei	Hopei Medical College (in Paoting)	Hopei Medical College (moved to Shihkiachwang)	Hopei College of New Medicine
	—	T'angshan Coal Mines Medical College [11]	Hopei Medical College
Hunan	Hunan Medical College (in Changsha)	Hunan Medical College	Hunan Medical College
Hupei	Hupei Medical College (in Wuchang, part of Wuhan)[12]	Hupei Medical College	Hupei Medical College
	Wuhan Medical College (in Hankow, part of Wuhan)[12]	Wuhan Medical College	Wuhan Medical College
Kansu	Lanchow Medical College	Lanchow Medical College	Lanchow Medical College
Kiangsi	Kiangsi Medical College (in Nanchang)	Kiangsi Medical College	Kiangsi Medical College
Kiangsu	Kiangsu Medical College (in Nanking)	Nanking Medical College	Kiangsu College of New Medicine (combining Nanking Medical College and Nanking Chinese Medical College)
	—	Nanking Chinese Medical College	
	Nanking College of Pharmacology	Nanking Pharmaceutical College	Nanking Pharmaceutical College
	—	Nanking Railway Medical College	Nanking Railway Medical College

Provinces[10]	1957	1964	1972
	—	Soochow Medical College	Soochow Medical College
	Nantung Medical College		Nantung Medical College
Kirin	Yenpien University Medical College (in Yenchi)	Kirin Medical University	Kirin Medical University [13]
	—	—	No information
		Changchun Medical College	No information
Kwangtung	Kwangchow (Canton) Medical College	Chungshan (Dr. Sun Yat-sen) Medical College	Chungshan Medical College
	Canton College of Chinese Medicine	Canton Chinese Medical College	Kwangchow College of Traditional Chinese Medicine
Kweichow	Kweiyang Medical College	Kweiyang Medical College	Kweiyang Medical College
	Chungking Medical College (possibly in Kweiyang)	—	No information
	—	—	Tsunyi Medical College [14]
Liaoning	Shenyang Medical College	Shenyang Medical College China Medical University (in Shenyang)	Shenyang Medical College (combining Shenyang Medical College and China Medical University)
	—		
	Dairen Medical College	Dairen Medical College	(Moved to Kweichow Province)[14]

Province			
	—	Shenyang Pharmaceutical College	Shenyang College of Traditional Chinese Medicine [15]
	Shenyang College of Pharmacology	—	Shenyang Pharmaceutical College
	—	—	Chinchow Medical College
Shansi	Shansi Medical College (in Taiyuan)	Shansi Medical College	Shansi Medical College
Shantung	Shantung Medical College (in Tsinan)	Shantung Medical College	Shantung Medical College [16]
	Tsingtao Medical College	Tsingtao Medical College	Tsingtao Medical College
	—	Shantung Chinese Medical College	Shantung College of Traditional Chinese Medicine [17]
Shensi	Sian Medical College	Sian Medical College	Sian Medical College
	—	Sian Military Medical University	Sian Military Medical University [5]
Szechwan	Szechwan Medical College (in Chengtu)	Szechwan Medical College	Szechwan Medical College
	Chungking Medical College	Chungking Medical College	Chungking Medical College
	Chengtu College of Chinese Medicine	Chengtu Chinese Medical College	Chengtu College of Traditional Chinese Medicine

Provinces [10]	1957	1964	1972
Tsinghai	—	—	Tsinghai Medical College (in Sining)
Yunnan	Kunming Medical College	Kunming Chinese Medical College	Kunming Medical College / Yunnan College of Traditional Chinese Medicine

Autonomous Regions	1961	1964	1972
Inner Mongolia	Inner Mongolia Medical College (in Huhehot)	Inner Mongolia Medical College	Inner Mongolia Medical College
Kwangsi	Kwangsi Medical College (in Nanning)	Kwangsi Medical College	Kwangsi Medical College
Ningsia	—	—	Ningsia Medical College (in Yinchwan)
Sinkiang	Sinkiang Medical College (in Urumchi)	Sinkiang Medical College	Sinkiang Medical College
Tibet	—	—	None [18]

NOTES

1. Translated in *Current Background*, Hong Kong, U.S. Consulate General, no. 462 (July 1, 1957), from a brochure issued in March 1957 by the Chinese Ministry of Higher Education entitled "Guide to Institutions of Higher Education"; cited in Leo A. Orleans, *Professional Manpower and Education in Communist China* (Washington, D.C.: National Science Foundation, 1961): pp. 190-92.

2. *Management Organization and Structure of the Chinese Economy* (Tokyo: December 1964), cited in Leo A. Orleans, "Medical Education and Manpower in Communist China," in *Aspects of Chinese Education*, ed. C. T. Hu (New York: Columbia University Teachers College Press, 1969): p. 25.

3. Compiled from colleges mentioned to us by our hosts in 1971 and 1972; the list was reviewed and corrected by representatives of the Chinese Medical Association in 1972.

4. Several of our hosts referred to this school, which we visited in 1971 and 1972, as Peking First Medical College; the *Chinese Medical Journal* in 1973 refers to it as the Peking Medical College, the form used throughout this book.

5. Chan Chi-Chao, a medical student at the Chungshan Medical School from 1961 to 1967, and now a student at the Johns Hopkins University School of Medicine, states that "there are at least four military medical schools with six-year programs," (*Journal of Medical Education* 47 [1972]: 327-32). The only schools specifically identified by our hosts in 1972 were those in Shanghai and Sian.

6. A school whose name is variously translated as the China Medical University, Chinese People's Medical University, China Medical College, and Chinese Medical College was founded in 1959 as the successor to the Peking Union Medical College. It was an eight-year medical school, in contrast to the other five- or six-year schools. It is said to have ceased functioning as a medical school in the wake of the Cultural Revolution, but the Peking Union Medical College Hospital continues, as the Shoutu Hospital, to provide postgraduate and nursing education.

7. The Peking Second Medical College admitted its first class in 1972; its teaching hospitals are the Youyi, Gong-Nong-Bing, Chaoyang, and Children's.

8. The Shu Kuang Hospital of this college was cited as the source of an article in the *Chinese Medical Journal* no. 3 (March 1973): 32.

9. There was disagreement among our hosts about the extent to which the school, a part of China's national railway system, is still functioning.

10. Twenty-one provinces are listed; our hosts, however, referred to Taiwan as the PRC's "twenty-second" and "as yet unliberated" province.

11. The founding of this school, "China's first medical college for the training of medical doctors for coal mines," at the site of the K'ailan coal mining center in north China, was described in the *Chinese Medical Journal* 83 (1964): 270.

12. Wuhan is a "triple" city, consisting of Hankow, Hanyang, and Wuchang.

13. Cited as the source of an article in *Renmin Ribao (People's Daily)* (July 8, 1969), trans. in *Survey of China Mainland Press* no. 4459 (July 22, 1969).

14. Our hosts told us that the former Dairen Medical College had been moved, with its faculty and equipment, to Tsunyi in Kweichow Province.

15. Not mentioned during our visits, but visited by the delegation to China from the Institute of Medicine of the National Academy of Sciences in June 1973.

16. The philosophy represented by the leading body of this college during the Cultural Revolution is presented in

Revolutionary Committee of the "June 26th" Commune of the Shantung Medical College, "A New Approach to Medical Education," *China's Medicine* no. 5 (May 1968): 292-96.

17. Not mentioned during our visit but cited as the source of an article in *China's Medicine* no. 1 (January 1968): 54-64, and of an article in *Renmin Ribao* (July 8, 1969), trans. in *Survey of China Mainland Press* no. 4459 (July 22, 1969).

18. Our hosts stated that every province, independent city, and autonomous region, with the exception of Tibet, now has at least one medical college.

Note: A *World Directory of Medical Schools 1970* was published by the World Health Organization in 1973. Several of the schools mentioned to us in China in 1971 and 1972 are not included in the directory: for example, the Peking Second Medical College, the Shanghai Railway Medical College, and the military medical colleges. Conversely, some of the colleges in the directory were not listed for us: for example, medical colleges in Wenchow (Chekiang Province), Kiamusze (Heilungkiang), and Weifang (Shantung); and colleges of traditional Chinese medicine in Harbin (Heilungkiang), Changsha (Hunan), Wuhan (Hupei), Kweiyang (Kweichow), Sian (Shensi), and Nanning (Kwangsi Autonomous Region).

Description of an Electrostimulator Used in Acupuncture Treatment and Anesthesia

Bryan Parker, Seymour Furman, and Victor W. Sidel *

Acupuncture is a diagnostic and therapeutic technique with a recorded history of 2,000 years and a legendary history of 3,500 years. As part of the attempt by the People's Republic of China to combine traditional medical practices with Western-style medicine, many old uses for acupuncture are being reexplored, and many new uses for the technique are being developed. In several recent experimental therapeutic applications, electrical stimulation is being applied to the acupuncture needles.

Another new use of acupuncture that has captured much attention in the West is in providing anesthesia during surgery. American visitors to the PRC have witnessed and have reported on a number of major operations under acupuncture anesthesia. Some of these were done by electrostimulation of the acupuncture needle and others by manual manipulation of the needle. Sidel brought back an example, purchased in a medical equipment shop in Peking, of one type of electrostimulator used to produce anesthesia. The instrument was subjected to testing in the electronics laboratory of the Montefiore Hospital and Medical Center.

DESCRIPTION OF THE INSTRUMENT

The electrostimulator shown in Figure 22 is approximately five inches long, three inches wide, and one-and-one-half inches deep. It is labeled "Worker, Peasant and Soldier Electrostimulator Model Number Three." The label also reads "First National

* Mr. Parker is the director of the Bioengineering Department at the Montefiore Hospital and Medical Center; Dr. Furman is a member of the Department of Surgery at Montefiore Hospital and Medical Center and associate professor of surgery at the Albert Einstein College of Medicine.

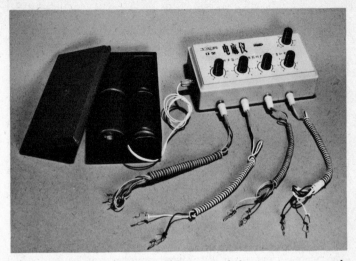

FIGURE 22. Electrostimulator with external battery power supply.

Peking Electrical Factory, May 7th Workers' School." * The circuit diagram for the stimulator, supplied in the accompanying instruction manual and confirmed by the authors, is shown in Figure 23.

A separate battery pack, also shown in Figure 22, may be used with the stimulator. It too is manufactured in Peking and is apparently a general purpose, remote battery pack that may also be used for transistor radios. Four 1.5 v. cells (equivalent in size to our D cells) are used in series in the battery pack, supplying a 6-v. output through a male jack. The electrostimulator also has provision for an internal 6-v. battery. The battery supplied with the stimulator was manufactured in Shanghai and has an output of 6 v.; it has no United States equivalent.

* The reference to a May 7th school on the instrument face indicates that it was produced as part of the program, initiated since the Great Proletarian Cultural Revolution, whereby intellectuals participate in physical labor in either communes or factories. May 7th schools have been established in a number of locations, and cadres (political workers), managers, teachers, and other "intellectuals" are rotated through them.

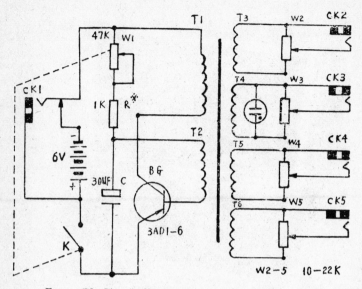

FIGURE 23. Circuit diagram from instruction manual.

A set of twenty-seven stainless steel acupuncture needles, presented to Sidel by the Chinese Medical Association, is shown in Figure 24. The overall length of the smallest needle is 3.8 cm. and that of the longest, 13.8 cm. Needles shorter than 9 cm. are 0.03 cm. in diameter, and consequently have a surface area of 0.1 cm.² per cm. of length. The longer electrodes have a diameter of 0.046 cm. Copper wire is wrapped around 2 to 3 cm. of the proximal end of the stainless steel needle, increasing the diameter to 0.11 cm., presumably to facilitate manipulation and/or electrical contact.

The stimulator produces a pulse which, measured across a 500-ohm load, has a duration of 1.94 msec. There are four individual outputs, the voltage of each individually controllable through a potentiometer. The voltage across a 500-ohm load at each potentiometer setting is shown in Table 19.

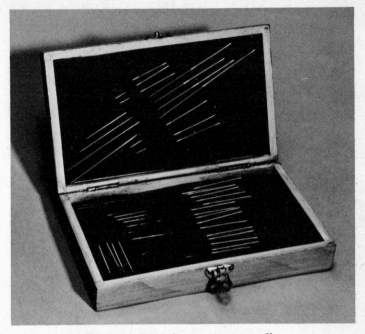

FIGURE 24. Box of acupuncture needles.

TABLE 19. VOLTAGE PRODUCED AT VARIOUS SETTINGS *

Dial Setting	Volts
0	0
1	1.25
2	2.0
3	3.5
4	6.5
5	stops

* Measured across a 500-ohm load.

Another potentiometer controls the on-off switch and determines the frequency of the pulses. Table 20 shows the number of pulses per minute at each dial setting. The wave form for a train of pulses at voltage setting 2, frequency setting 5, is shown in Figure 25.

The electrical characteristics of the needles can be inferred from the voltage and current waveforms shown in Figure 26, which were obtained with 2.4 cm. of a 5.4 cm.-long needle inserted in the thoracic musculature of an anesthetized dog. The other connection to the tissue was a large, subcutaneous, stainless steel plate about 10 cm. distant. At potentiometer setting 3, peak current flow was 7.5 mamps., and the applied voltage was 3.6 v., representing a load of 480 ohms. At maximum output setting of the stimulator, the peak current was 50 mamps. at

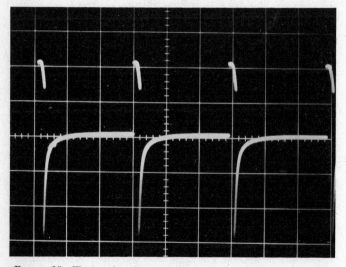

FIGURE 25. Train of pulses, voltage setting 2, frequency setting 5, 500-ohm load, 2 mamp. per vertical division, 10 msec. per horizontal division.

TABLE 20. RATE OF PULSATION AT VARIOUS SETTINGS *

Dial Setting	Pulses/min.
Minimum	77.3
1	77.3
2	87.5
3	137.0
4	314.0
5	2000.0

* Measured across a 500-ohm load.

17 v.; consequently the load was 340 ohms. The inverse relationship between load and current flow is usual with physiologic electrodes. Current was also introduced via two needles about 5 cm. apart, both similar in size and inserted in a similar way to the needle described above. At potentiometer setting 3, the peak current flow was 5.7 mamps. and the resistance 1,300 ohms. The waveforms for this configuration are shown in Figure 27.

INSTRUCTION MANUAL

Accompanying the instrument is a small instruction manual * whose cover reads "Electronic Device Instruction Book." On the inside front cover appear several sayings of Chairman Mao Tse-tung, and pages 1-6 contain additional inspirational material.

Pages 6-11 read:

Circuit Principles:

This instrument comprises a high-power, low-frequency transistor type BG, which, together with the resistance R and the capacitor C and the transformer, acts as a blocking oscillator. The variable resistor W1 controls the frequency of oscillation. The transformer also steps up the impulse voltage and connects it to four independently isolated pairs of wires. The strength of the output is adjusted by resistors W2, W3, W4, and W5.

A neon tube is connected across W3 and serves to check the instrument function. The circuit diagram is in the appendix.

* We are grateful to Dr. Tai H. Pan of the Department of Anesthesia, Montefiore Hospital, for his translation of portions of the instruction manual.

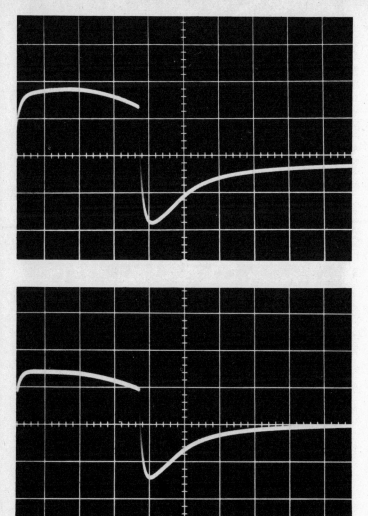

FIGURE 26. Voltage and current waveform with stimulator attached to acupuncture needles and subcutaneous plate, voltage setting 3, 0.5 msec. per horizontal division. Top: Voltage waveform 2v./div.; bottom: current waveform, 5 mamp./div.

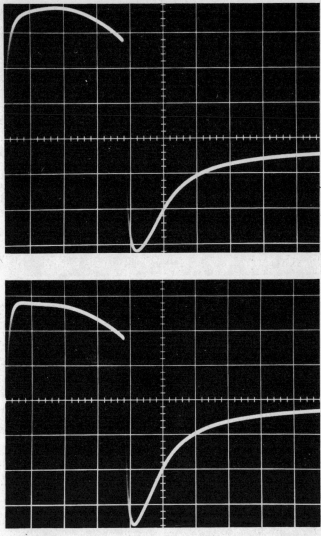

FIGURE 27. Voltage and current waveform with stimulator attached to two acupuncture needles, voltage setting 3, 0.5 msec. per horizontal division. Top: Voltage waveform, 2 v./div.; bottom: current waveform, 2 mamp./div.

Main technical characteristics:

1. Type of wave: A positive square wave with a negative overswing.
2. Width of wave: 500-1000 μsec.
3. Output voltage: approximately 90v.
4. Frequency: 1.5 to 40 pulses/sec.
5. Size: $139 \times 71 \times 39$ mm.
6. Weight: approximately 400 g.
7. Power requirement: 6v.

Method of Use:

1. Turn upper right hand knob clockwise from "OFF". The neon light should flash to indicate that the instrument is working normally.
2. Four adjustable knobs on the lower front panel adjust the strength of the four outputs. Before surgery or therapy, insert the four connectors into the jacks in the instrument. Firmly clench each wire pair in the hand. Adjust the output knobs from zero clockwise to the right. The fingers will feel vibrations from weak to strong. Check each knob to be sure that output is normal; then turn all knobs to the zero position. (Because of variations in skin moisture individual differences in sensation will occur. If necessary moisten the hand with water.)
3. There are two wires from each plug; the red is positive and the other color is negative. Connect wires to the tips of the acupuncture needles. Then adjust the output knob to control the strength of the electric current.
4. Vary the rate, strength of output and frequency, and duration of treatment as indicated by the progress of the operation or therapy.
5. During therapy wet cotton combined with electrodes may be used on the surface of the body to increase stimulation.
6. After use turn the rate knob to OFF, turn each output control to zero, and disconnect the needles.

Caution

1. After connection to the body, loading may reduce the voltage to the point where the neon lamp ceases to flash. This is normal and does not influence usage of the instrument.
2. After using the instrument remove the plug from the auxiliary battery pack. Put the plastic cover over the plug. Otherwise an accidental short circuit may discharge the battery.
3. There is a 6v. battery within the instrument. If an external

TABLE 21. STATISTICS OF ACUPUNCTURE USE IN ANESTHESIA IN XIANGYANG HOSPITAL, PEKING

Procedure	Number of Cases	Result				Method			Comment
		A	B	C	D	M	E	S	
Appendectomy	5	4	1				X		
Hernia repair	6	2	4				X		
Thyroidectomy (tumor)	2	2					X		One case combination of mechanical and electrical
Thyroidectomy (cyst)	2	2					X		
Acute perforation of stomach	2	2				X			
Hip pinning	1	1					X		Only one case with excellent results
Tumor removal from hip	1	1					X		
Mastectomy	2	2					X		
Hydrocelectomy	1		1				X		
Orchiectomy	1		1				X		
Laparotomy	1		1			X			
Removal of pelvic tumor	1				1		X		
Hemorrhoidectomy	1		1				X		
Tubal ligation	13	7	6				X		One case has electrically positive site
Cesarian section	5	5				X			One case manual technique and electrical
Ovarian cystectomy	3	2	1				X		

					S
Subtotal hysterectomy	2			2	X
Total hysterectomy	1			1	X
Eye	1	1			X
Tooth	2	2			X
Total	53	33	19	1	

Result code: A-excellent; B-good; C-fair; D-failure; method code: M-mechanical; E-electrical; S-site.

battery pack is used or if the instrument is not to be used for some time remove the internal battery. This will prevent corrosion which could destroy the instrument.

4. If the voltage from the external or internal battery is low the strength of stimulation will decrease. If the neon light does not flash install a new battery. The internal battery is Model 4F45-2 6v. (made in Shanghai). The remote battery has four Size 1 cells (available at any shop).

Pages 12-16 are entitled "Mao Tse-tung's Thought Illuminates the Work of Acupuncture in Our Hospital." Pages 17-20 provide some statistics on the use of the instrument in anesthesia at Xiangyang Hospital in Peking (Table 21).

DISCUSSION

The stimulator seems to be simple and well-designed. The 2 msec. pulse duration suggests that it was intended for both nerve and muscle stimulation rather than primarily for nerve stimulation, or at least that would be its use in the United States. One or two of the components seem identical to components made in Japan, but there is no indication that they were made elsewhere than in China; all components identified as to place of manufacture are labeled as having been made in the PRC.

The mechanism of action of acupuncture anesthesia is as yet unknown, as is the role of electrostimulation in it. The only thing that can be stated at present is that all who have observed surgery under acupuncture anesthesia agree that it indeed appears to work successfully on the patients whose operations they witnessed. The phenomenon is therefore clearly of practical as well as of theoretical interest to us in the United States.

NOTE

An analysis of a different type of stimulator used in China was published in July 1973, after the completion of this report. See A.M. Basich, "An Analysis of a Portable Electronic Stimulator Manufactured in the People's Republic of China," *American Journal of Chinese Medicine* 1 (July 1973):341-50.

Institutes of the Chinese Academy
of Medical Sciences

1961 LISTING *

Located in Peking

Institute of Acupuncture and Moxibustion
Institute of Antibiotics
Institute of Biological Products
Institute of Blood Transfusion and Hemopathology
Institute of Dermatology
Institute of Epidemiology and Microbiology
Institute of Hypertension
Institute of Internal Medicine
Laboratory of Isotopes
Institute of Labor Hygiene, Labor Protection, and Occupational Diseases
Institute of Medical Radiology
Institute of Microbiology
Institute of Oncology
Institute of Parasitology
Institute of Pediatrics
Institute of Pharmacology
Institute of Surgery
Institute of Traditional Chinese Drugs
Institute of Tuberculosis

Located in Fukien

Institute of Epidemiology, Amoy
Institute of Epidemiology, Foochow

* Source: Leo Orleans, *Professional Manpower and Education in Communist China* (Washington, D.C.: Government Printing Office, 1961): p. 245.

Located in Shensi

   Institute of Acupuncture and Moxibustion, Sian
   Institute of Traditional Chinese Medicine, Sian

1972 LISTING *

Located in Peking

   Institute of Cardiovascular Disease
   Institute of Epidemiological Research (includes former Institute of Virology)
   Institute of Experimental Medicine
   Institute of Health (Institute of Industrial Hygiene)[1]
   Institute of Hematologic Diseases
   Institute of Medical Biology (includes former Institute of Antibiotics)
   Institute of Materia Medica
   Tumor Institute (Institute of Cancer Research)[2]

Located in Shanghai [3]

   Institute of Parasitic Diseases
   Institute for Materia Medica

Located in Kiangsu

   Institute of Dermatology

* Source: Compiled from institutes mentioned to us by our hosts in 1971 and 1972, and reviewed in 1972 by representatives of the CMA; the list is probably incomplete. In addition to the institutes of CAMS, there are research institutes associated with the Academy of Traditional Chinese Medicine and with the Chinese Academy of Sciences, which are separate organizations.

NOTES

1. The Institute of Health, and its divisions of occupational health and of environmental health, were cited as sources of articles in the *Chinese Medical Journal* in 1973. An "Institute of Industrial Hygiene," mentioned by our hosts, is probably the same institute.

2. The Tumor Institute was cited in the February 1973 issue of the *Chinese Medical Journal.* An "Institute of Cancer Research" mentioned by our hosts is probably the same institute. It appears to be very closely associated with the Jih Tan Hospital of CAMS.

3. Other research institutes located in Shanghai, but apparently not part of CAMS, are the Research Institute of Cardiovascular Diseases and the Institute of Physiology; these are cited as sources of articles in the *Chinese Medical Journal* in 1973.

Acknowledgments

The number of people and institutions to whom we are indebted for advice and help in the course of our visits to China, as well as in the preparation of the reports on it, is almost endless. One of the greatest joys of this experience has been people both in the East and in the West whom we met and with whom we worked.

Among those who have been most helpful are Professor Arthur Galston of Yale University, whose recommendation of us to Dr. Kuo Mo-jo led to our invitation to visit China, and who has provided counsel both before and since our visits; Comrades Chang Wei-hsun, Hong Ming-gui, Hsieh Hua, Hsu Shou-jen, Li Chun-hen, Liu Kuei, Ma Hai-teh, Hans Muller, and Young Ming-ting of the People's Republic of China, whose warmth, generosity, and patience were unique in our experience and can never be repaid; Hsu Chia-yu, whose indefatigable interpretation of his country to us during both our visits to China and during his visit here has been indispensable to our understanding; members of the Mission of the People's Republic of China to the United Nations for clarification of a number of points; Dr. Martin Cherkasky, Director of Montefiore Hospital, for his constant encouragement; Dr. John Z. Bowers of the Macy Foundation, who generously shared his knowledge of medicine in China and suggested, supported, and commented on the manuscript of this report; Shirley Schwartz for her editorial assistance with an early version of the report; Janice Kaplan, Dinah Reitman, and Susan Weinstein for their help with the references and bibliography; Livia Cersosimo, Marianne Kennedy, Terry Miller,

Sharon Patterson, Eve Teitelbaum, and Sara Wolk for typing portions of the manuscript; Mark Sidel who contributed Appendix D; Steven Lamm who collaborated on Appendix E; Bryan Parker and Seymour Furman who collaborated on Appendix J; Estelle Holt, Daniel Drosness, and Ernest Drucker of the Department of Social Medicine of Montefiore Hospital who kept its work going so this could be written; and Kevin Sidel whose good cheer urged us on.

Portions of the material in this book have been used by one or both of us, in other forms and often in greater detail, in articles that have already appeared or are in press in the *American Journal of Orthopsychiatry, Asia, Human Behavior, International Journal of Health Services, New England Journal of Medicine, New Physician, Proceedings of the Academy of Political Science, Social Policy,* and *Social Work,* in chapters in the books, *China Medicine As We Saw It* (Fogarty International Center), *Medicine and Public Health in the People's Republic of China* (Fogarty International Center), *National Health Services* (Macy Foundation) and *Public Health in the People's Republic of China* (Macy Foundation), and in *Women and Child Care in China* (Hill and Wang). Specific citations for those already published may be found in the bibliography. We are grateful to the editors and publishers of these journals and books for giving us the opportunity to help disseminate information on medical care in China as widely as possible.

Special thanks are due to Elizabeth Purcell of the Macy Foundation for her patience and skill in editing this report.

Bibliography

I. CHINA PRIOR TO 1949

A. General

Belden, Jack. *China Shakes the World.* New York: Monthly Review Press, 1949 (Reprint ed., paperback, 1970).

Ch'en, Jerome. *Mao and the Chinese Revolution.* London: Oxford University Press, 1965 (Reprint ed., with corrections, 1970).

Hinton, William. *Fanshen: A Documentary of Revolution in a Chinese Village.* New York: Random House, Vintage Books, paperback, 1966.

Pruitt, Ida. *A Daughter of Han: The Autobiography of A Chinese Working Woman.* New Haven: Yale University Press, 1945.

Russell, Bertrand. *The Problem of China.* London: George Allen and Unwin, 1922 (Reprint ed., 1972).

Snow, Edgar. *Red Star Over China.* New York: Random House, 1938.

Thomson, James C., Jr. *While China Faced West.* Cambridge: Harvard University Press, 1969.

White, Theodore H., and Jacoby, Annalee. *Thunder Out of China*. New York: William Sloan, 1946 (reprint ed., 1973).

B. Medicine

Allen, Ted, and Gordon, Sydney. *The Scalpel, The Sword.* Boston: Little-Brown, 1952 (Rev. ed., paperback, Toronto: McClelland and Stewart, 1971).

Bowers, John Z. *Western Medicine in a Chinese Palace: Peking Union Medical College, 1917-1951*. New York: Josiah Macy, Jr. Foundation, 1973.

Ferguson, Mary E. *China Medical Board and Peking Union Medical College. A Chronicle of Fruitful Collaboration, 1914-1951*. New York: China Medical Board of New York, 1970.

Hume, Edward H. *Doctors East Doctors West: An American Physician's Life in China*. New York: Norton, 1946.

Lamson, Herbert Day. *Social Pathology in China*. Shanghai: The Commercial Press, 1935.

Needham, Joseph. *The Grand Titration: Science and Society in East and West*. London: George Allen and Unwin, 1969.

Sze, Szeming. *China's Health Problems*. Washington, D.C.: Chinese Medical Association, 1943.

C. English-Language Medical Journals Published in China

China Medical Missionary Journal. Published by the China Medical Missionary Association from 1887 to 1907, when title became the *China Medical Journal*.

China Medical Journal. Published by the China Medical Missionary Association (renamed the China Medical Association in 1925) from 1907 to 1931, when it was merged with *National Medical Journal of China* to form the *Chinese Medical Journal*.

National Medical Journal of China. Published by the National Medical Association of China from 1915 to 1931, when it was merged with the *China Medical Journal* to form the *Chinese Medical Journal*.

Chinese Medical Journal. Published by the Chinese Medical Association from January 1932.

II. CHINA SINCE 1949

A. From Liberation to Cultural Revolution

Greene, Felix. *Awakened China*. Garden City, N.Y.: Doubleday, 1961.

Han Suyin, "Reflections on Social Change." *Bulletin of the Atomic Scientists* 22, no. 6 (June 1966):80-33.

Karol, K. S. *China: The Other Communism*. New York: Hill and Wang, paperback, 1968.

Myrdal, Jan. *Report from a Chinese Village*. New York: New American Library, 1966.

Orleans, Leo A. *Professional Manpower and Education in Communist China*. Washington, D.C., Government Printing Office, 1961.

Schurmann, Franz. *Ideology and Organization in Communist China*. Berkeley: University of California Press, paperback 1973.

Snow, Edgar. *Red China Today*. New York: Random House, Vintage Books, paperback, 1971 (Rev. ed. of *The Other Side of the River*, published in 1962).

Solomon, Richard H. *Mao's Revolution and the Chinese Political Culture*. Berkeley: University of California Press, 1971.

B. The Cultural Revolution and Beyond

1. Books

Committee of Concerned Asia Scholars. *China! Inside the People's Republic*. New York: Bantam Books, 1972.

Durdin, Tillman, Reston, James, and Topping, Seymour. *Report from Red China*. New York: Quandrangle Books, 1971.

Hinton, William. *Hundred Day War: The Cultural Revolution at Tsinghua University*. New York: Monthly Review Press, paperback, 1972.

Joint Economic Committee, Congress of the United States. *People's Republic of China: An Economic Assessment*. Washington, D.C.: U.S. Government Printing Office, 1972.

Macciocchi, Maria Antonietta. *Daily Life in Revolutionary China*. New York: Monthly Review Press, 1972.

Oksenberg, Michel, ed. *China's Developmental Experience*. New York: Academy of Political Science, Columbia University, *Proceedings of the Academy of Political Science* 31, no. 1 (March 1973).

Robinson, Joan. *The Cultural Revolution in China*. Baltimore: Penguin Books, 1969.

Shabad, Theodore. *China's Changing Map*. New York: Praeger, paperback, 1972.

Sidel, Ruth. *Women and Child Care in China: A First-Hand Report*. New York: Hill and Wang, 1972.

Whitaker, Donald P., and Shinn, Rinn-Sup. *Area Handbook for the People's Republic of China*. Washington, D.C.: U.S. Government Printing Office, 1972.

2. Articles

Frolic, Michael B. "What the Cultural Revolution Was All About." *The New York Times Magazine* (October 24, 1971).

Galston, Arthur W. "The Chinese University." *Natural History* 81 (August-September, 1972):18, 20, 22-23.

———. "The University in China." *Bioscience* 22 (1972):217-20.

Gurley, John G. "Capitalist and Maoist Economic Development." In *America's Asia,* edited by Edward Freedman and Mark Selden. New York: Random House, Vintage Books, 1971.

Leontief, Wassily. "Socialism in China." *The Atlantic* 231, no. 3 (March 1973):74-81.

Lubkin, Gloria B. "Physics in China." *Physics Today* 25 (December 1972): 23-28.

Sidel, Ruth. "Social Services in China." *Social Work* 17 (November 1972): 5-13.

Sidel, Ruth, and Sidel, Victor W. "The Human Services in China." *Social Policy* 2 (March-April 1972):25-34.

Signer, Ethan. "Biological Science in China." *Science for the People* 3 (September 1971):3-5, 15-19.

Signer, Ethan, and Galston, Arthur W. "Education and Science in China." *Science* 175 (1972):15-19.

Tsu, Raphael. "High Technology in China." *Scientific American* 227 (December 1972):13-17.

Yang, Chen-ning. "C. N. Yang Discusses Physics in the People's Republic of China." *Physics Today* 24 (November 1971):61-63.

III. Medicine in China Since 1949

A. Overview

Cheng, Tien-Hsi. "Schistosomiasis in Mainland China: A Review of Research and Control Programs Since 1949." *American Journal of Tropical Medicine and Hygiene* 20 (1971):26-53.

Horn, Joshua S. *Away with All Pests . . . An English Surgeon in People's China, 1954-1969.* New York: Monthly Review Press, 1969 (Reprint ed., paperback, 1971).

Kao, Frederick F. "China, Chinese Medicine, and the Chinese Medical System." *American Journal of Chinese Medicine* 1, no. 1 (January 1973): 1-59.

Lampton, David M. "Public Health and Politics in China's Past Two Decades." *Health Services Reports* 87, no. 10 (December 1972):895-904.

Liang, Matthew H. et al. "Chinese Health Care: Determinants of the System." *American Journal of Public Health* 63 (1972):102-10.

Orleans, Leo A. *Every Fifth Child: The Population of China.* Stanford: Stanford University Press, 1972.

Selden, Mark. "China: Revolution and Health." *Health/PAC Bulletin* no. 47 (1972).

B. Pre-Cultural Revolution

Baltzan, David M., and Maddin, W. Stuart. "Medicine in China." *Canadian Medical Association Journal* 93 (1965):1118-22.

Best, J. B. "The Wider View: Impressions on a Recent Visit to China (April-May 1966)." *The Medical Journal of Australia* 2 (December 24, 1966):1242-47.

Chen, W. Y. "Medicine and Public Health in China Today." *Public Health Reports* 76 (1961):699-711.

Chinese Medical Journal. Published by the Chinese Medical Association through September 1966.

For the Health of the People. Peking: Foreign Languages Press, 1967.

Fox, Theodore. "The New China: Some Medical Impressions." *Lancet* 2 (1957):935-39, 955-99, 1053-57.

Lowinger, Paul. "How China Solved the Drug Problem." *Social Policy* 3, no. 2 (July-August 1972):11-43.

Orleans, Leo A. "Medical Education and Manpower in Communist China." In *Aspects of Chinese Education,* edited by C. T. Hu. New York: Columbia University Teachers College Press, 1969.

Pa Chin et al. *A Battle for Life: A Full Record of How the Life of Steel Worker Chiu Tsai-Fang Was Saved in the Shanghai Kwangtze Hospital.* Peking: Foreign Languages Press, 1959.

Penfield, Wilder. "Oriental Renaissance in Education and Medicine." *Science* 141 (1963):1153-61.

Worth, Robert M. "Health Trends in China Since the 'Great Leap Forward.'" *American Journal of Hygiene* 78 (1963):349-57.

—————. "Health in Rural China: From Village to Commune." *American Journal of Hygiene* 77 (1963):228-39.

C. Post-Cultural Revolution

1. Books and Special Issues of Journals

Brown, Maggie, ed. *Science and Medicine in the People's Republic of China. Asia* no. 26 (1972).

Medical Workers Serving the People Wholeheartedly. Peking: Foreign Languages Press, 1971.

National Medical Association China Visit Number. Special Issue, *Journal of National Medical Association* 65 no. 1 (January 1973):1-87.

Piotrow, Phyllis T., ed. *Population and Family Planning in the People's Republic of China.* Washington, D.C.: Victor-Bostrom Fund and the Population Crisis Committee, 1971.

Quinn, Joseph R., ed. *Medicine and Public Health in the People's Republic of China.* Department of Health, Education, and Welfare Publication No. (NIH) 72-67. Fogarty International Center, National Institutes of Health, Bethesda, Maryland, 1972.

Scaling Peaks in Medical Science. Peking: Foreign Languages Press, 1972.

Wegman, Myron E., Lin, Tsung-yi, and Purcell, Elizabeth F., eds. *Public Health in the People's Republic of China.* New York: Josiah Macy, Jr. Foundation, 1973.

2. Articles

Aaron, Harold. "Notes on Drugs and Therapeutics in the People's Republic of China." *The Medical Letter* 14 (1972):65-68.

Bowers, John Z. "Medicine in Mainland China: Red and Rural." *Current Scene* 8 (1970):1-11.

Chan, Chi-chao. "Medical Education in Mainland China." *Journal of Medical Education* 47 (1972):327-32.

Cheng, T. O. "A View of Modern Chinese Medicine." *Annals of Internal Medicine* 78(1973):285-90.

"China Explains Her Views on the Population Question." *Peking Review* no. 17 (1973): 16-17.

"China's Family Planning: 'Stunning.'" *Medical World News* (May 18, 1973):50.

Dimond, E. Grey. "Medical Education and Care in People's Republic of China." *Journal of the American Medical Association* 218 (1971):1552-57.

———. "Medicine in the People's Republic of China: A Progress Report." *Journal of the American Medical Association* 222 (1972):1158-59.

———. "More than Herbs and Acupuncture." *Saturday Review* 54 (1971): 17-19.

Faundes, Anibal, and Luukkainen, Tapani. "Health and Family Planning Services in the Chinese People's Republic." *Studies in Family Planning* Supp. 3 (1972).

Flato, Charles. "The Medical Revolution." *Nation* 215 (1972):397-99.

Geiger, H. Jack. "Putting China's Medicine in Perspective." *Medical World News* 14, no. 20 (May 18, 1972):43-49.

———. "A Pragmatic Approach to Medicine." *Medical World News* 14, no. 23 (June 1, 1973):22-25.

Jain, K. K. "Glimpses of Chinese Medicine, 1971" *Canadian Medical Association Journal* 106 (1972): 46-50.

Kagan, Leigh. "Report from a Visit to the Tientsin Psychiatric Hospital, March 1972." *China Notes* 10 (1972):37-39.

"Medicine in China." *Medical World News* 13 (1972):51-58, 62.

Orleans, Leo A., and Suttmeier, R. P. "The Mao Ethic and Environmental Quality." *Science* 170 (1970):1173-76.

———. "China: Population in the People's Republic." *Population Bulletin* 27 (1971).

———. "China's Statistics: The System and Its Problems." *Public Data Use* 1 (1973):17-23.

Pickowicz, Paul G. "Barefoot Doctors in China: People, Politics and Paramedicine." *Eastern Horizon* 11 (1971):25-38.

Reyes, V. A. "A Brief Glimpse of Medicine in the People's Republic of China." *Journal of the Phillipine Medical Association* 43 (1967):385-98.

Rifkin, S. B. "Public Health in China: Is the Experience Relevant to

Other Less Developed Nations?" *Social Science and Medicine* 7 (1973): 249-57.

Robb, Sir Douglas. "Medicine in China." *New Zealand Medical Journal* 66 (1967):183-87.

Sidel, Ruth. "Women in Medicine in the People's Republic of China." *The New Physician* 22 (1973):300-305.

Sidel, Victor W. "Primary Care in the People's Republic of China." In *Milbank Memorial Fund Seminar Report—Mexico City, 1972.* New York: Milbank Memorial Fund (1972): pp. 34-40.

————. "Serve the People: Medical Education in the People's Republic of China." *The New Physician* 21 (1972):284-91.

————. "Some Observations on the Organization of Health Care in the People's Republic of China." *International Journal of Health Services* 2 (1972):385-95.

————. "The Barefoot Doctors of the People's Republic of China." *New England Journal of Medicine* 286 (1972):1292-99.

Stanley, Margaret. "Two Experiences of an American Public Health Nurse." *American Journal of Public Health* 63 (1973):111-16.

Thomason, R. K. C., MacKenzie, W. C., and Pert, A. F. W. "A Visit to the People's Republic of China." *Canadian Medical Association Journal* 97 (1967):349-60.

White, Paul D. "China's Heart Is in the Right Place." *New York Times* (December 5, 1971).

Worth, Robert M. "Strategy of Change in the People's Republic of China— The Rural Health Center." In *Communication and Change in the Developing Countries,* edited by D. Lerner and W. Schramm. Eastwood Center, 1971.

3. English-Language Medical Journals Published in China

China's Medicine. (Published by the Chinese Medical Association from October 1966 through December 1968).

Chinese Medical Journal. (Published by the CMA beginning in January 1973).

IV. TRADITIONAL CHINESE MEDICINE

1. Books

Acupuncture Anesthesia. Peking: Foreign Languages Press, 1972.

Beau, Georges. *Chinese Medicine.* New York: Avon Books, paperback, 1972.

Croizier, Ralph C. *Traditional Medicine in Modern China.* Cambridge: Harvard University Press, 1968.

Duke, Marc. *Acupuncture.* New York: Pyramid House, 1972.

Exploring the Secrets of Treating Deaf-Mutes. Peking: Foreign Languages Press, 1972.

Huard, Pierre, and Wong, Ming. *Chinese Medicine*. London: World University Library, paperback, 1968.

Mann, Felix. *Acupuncture: The Ancient Chinese Art of Healing*. New York: Random House, 1962 (Reprint ed., paperback, Vintage Books, 1972).

Monaka, Yoshio, and Urquhart, Ian A. *The Layman's Guide to Acupuncture*. New York: John Weatherhill, 1972.

Moss, Louis. *Acupuncture and You*. New York: Citadel Press, 1964.

Palos, Stephan. *The Chinese Art of Healing*. Translation by Translagency, Ltd. New York: Herder and Herder, 1971 (Reprint ed., paperback, Bantam Books, 1972).

Tan, Leong C., Tan, Margaret Y. C., and Veith, Ilza. *Acupuncture Therapy: Current Chinese Practice*. Philadelphia: Temple University Press, 1973.

Veith, Ilza, trans. *Huang-ti Nei-ching Su-wen (The Yellow Emperor's Classic of Internal Medicine)*. Berkeley: University of California Press, 1972.

Wallnöfer, Heinrich, and Von Rottauscher, Anna. *Chinese Folk Medicine*. New York: Crown Publishers, 1965 (Reprint ed., paperback, New American Library, 1972).

2. Articles

Brown, P. E. "Use of Acupuncture in Major Surgery." *Lancet* 1 (1972) 1328-30.

Copperauld, I. "Acupuncture Anesthesia and Medicine in China Today." *Surgery, Gynecology, and Obstetrics* 135 (1972): 440-45.

Dimond, E. Grey. "Acupuncture Anesthesia: Western Medicine and Chinese Traditional Medicine." *Journal of the American Medical Association* 218 (1971):1558-63.

Galston, Arthur W. "Attitudes on Acupuncture 1971," *Yale Review* 61 (1972):312-17.

Geiger, H. Jack. "How Acupuncture Anesthetizes: The Chinese Explanation." *Medical World News* 14, no. 27 (July 13, 1973):51-61.

Halter, Jr., John S. "Acupuncture in Nineteenth Century Medicine." *New York State Journal of Medicine* 73 (1973):1213-21.

Melzack, Ronald. "How Acupuncture Works: A Sophisticated Western Theory Takes the Mystery Out." *Psychology Today* 7, no. 6 (June 1973):28-35.

Rosen, Samuel. "I Have Seen the Past and It Works." *New York Times* (November 1, 1971).

Veith, Ilza. "Acupuncture Therapy, Past and Present: Verity or Delusion." *Journal of the American Medical Association* 180 (1962):478-84.

V. CHINESE LANGUAGE

A Bibliography of Chinese Sources on Medicine and Public Health in the People's Republic of China: 1960-1970. Department of Health, Education, and Welfare Publication No. (NIH) 73-439. Fogarty International Center, National Institutes of Health, Bethesda, Maryland, 1972.

Chinese-English Dictionary . . . of Modern Communist Chinese Usage. 2nd ed. JPRS-20904. Washington, D.C.: Joint Publications Research Service, n.d. (Translation of a Chinese-German dictionary published in Peking in 1960 with romanization in *pinyin,* and conversion tables between the Wade-Giles system and *pinyin*).

Huang, C. C. *A Modern Chinese-English Dictionary for Students.* Lawrence: University of Kansas Center for Asian Studies, 1968 (A dictionary with romanization in *pinyin*).

Newnham, Richard. *About Chinese.* Baltimore: Penguin Books, paperback, 1971.

Wang, William S.Y. "The Chinese Language." *Scientific American* 228 (February 1973):50-63.

VI. Sources of Current Information in English Published
in China on a Regular Basis

China Pictorial (monthly)
China Reconstructs (monthly)
Chinese Medical Journal (monthly)
Peking Review (weekly)
(Subscriptions to these journals are available through Guozi Shudian, China Publications Center, P.O. Box 399, Peking, People's Republic of China.)

Index